Praise for *The Minimum Method*

"Joey Thurman is one of the clear, bright, consistent voices in the clouded landscape of wellness and fitness. In *The Minimum Method*, he brilliantly distills years of research, practice, and life lessons into a simple guide that can be an instant gamechanger for so many who need it."

—Ian K. Smith, MD, #1 *New York Times* bestselling author of *The Met Flex Diet*

"Joey has a gift. He is so in tune with the body and so knowledgeable he gets you to where you want or need to be in the most effective and efficient way. His keen eye was able to spot an oncoming injury I'd been trying to work around for years before the medical professionals by just being attentive. He was able to give me the tools I needed to balance, strengthen, and heal!"

—Wunmi Mosaku, award-winning actress

"Joey is a walking example of a healthy, well-balanced, active, and mindful lifestyle. He delivers a holistic approach to diet and exercise that is virtually foolproof for attaining good health . . . He understands the importance of individualization. Here's one of my favorite lines in the book, one of many memorable lessons that rings true: 'Information is rarely black-and-white—that's as much true for health and wellness as it is for anything else. So I give you permission to find your gray.'"

—Alan Aragon, nutrition researcher and leader of the evidence-based fitness movement

"Joey has made it easy to keep up with my fitness and hit my personal health goals while on the road touring, in and out of hotels, and going from town to town. He practices what he preaches with a deep knowledge and passion for lifestyle, nutrition, and fitness. He understands we are all different and addresses the needs of the masses while understanding individuality and preparing you for future success with your health and wellness mentally and physically."

—Michael Ray, multi-platinum country artist

"I've had the pleasure of learning from Joey for a while now, and I can honestly say he is one of the best. He pointed out things in my workouts that make the moves so much more efficient and effective. I highly recommend this book . . . and anything else he has to share!"

—Cameron Mathison, Emmy-nominated actor, Emmy-winning TV host

"Joey and his words are a testament to the perseverance of the human spirit and just how much can change when you show up for yourself (and for others)—even if some days that doesn't feel like much. He reminds us that you don't have to be superhuman every single day to change yourself or the world."

—Laura Micetich, the Iron Giantess

"I've been working out for more than twenty years and every time I've trained with Joey my limits have always been tested! From diet and exercise to recovery—especially when coming back from my ACL replacement. I trust his knowledge and would recommend him to beginners, athletes, and trainers alike."

—Mickie James-Aldis, 10-times women's wrestling champion, singer/songwriter

"Joey combines science with a relatable, minimalistic approach and it's the fitness equation I've been waiting for. No gimmicks, no frills. Sign me up."

—Dr. Alok Patel, ABC News special correspondent,
cohost of PBS's *Parentalogic*, and host of *NOVA Now*

THE MINIMUM METHOD

THE MINIMUM METHOD

The Least You Can Do to Be a Stronger, Healthier, Happier You

JOEY THURMAN

FOREWORD BY DR. WILL COLE

BenBella Books, Inc.
Dallas, TX

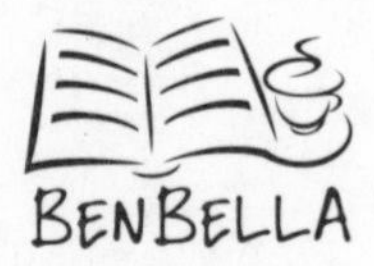

BenBella Books, Inc.
10440 N. Central Expressway
Suite 800
Dallas, TX 75231
benbellabooks.com
Send feedback to feedback@benbellabooks.com

BenBella is a federally registered trademark.

Printed in the United States of America
10 9 8 7 6 5 4 3 2 1

Library of Congress Control Number: 2022024692
ISBN 9781637742297 (hardcover)
ISBN 9781637742303 (electronic)

Editing by Ruth Strother
Proofreading by Madeline Grigg and Isabelle Rubio
Indexing by WordCo Indexing Services, Inc.
Text design and composition by PerfecType, Nashville, TN
Interior illustrations by Frankie Martinelli
Cover design by Oceana Garceau
Cover images © Shutterstock / Semanche (man with salad), Shutterstock / NatalieZhy (woman in chair), Shutterstock / Amaro_K (check mark), and iStock / A-Digit(yoga figure; meditation figure)
Printed by Lake Book Manufacturing

For my son.

May all of your dreams come true, your light stay bright, your heart be full of love, and you never forget the answer to my question, "What is the favorite part of my day?"

Contents

Foreword

In today's world, saturated with fad diets, aggressive exercise regimens, and incredibly unrealistic body standards, it's hard to know with certainty how to get and stay healthy. The sheer amount of (often competing) information out there makes it extremely difficult to separate fact from fiction.

This is where Joey Thurman—a health, fitness, and nutrition expert—comes in to help. He's done the research and translated it into something all of us can understand and apply. Most importantly though, Joey acknowledges that the messages the fitness world often sends are both unrealistic and deeply unhealthy. As an insider in the exercise and health industry, Joey knows firsthand how harmful the effects of a "go, go, go" and "push your limits all day, every day" lifestyle can be on our collective health—physically, mentally, and emotionally.

The Minimum Method is a refreshing reexamination of fitness with useful and practical advice on how to stay healthy with minimum effort, just like the title says. A lot of people simply don't have the time, energy, or resources to follow dramatic fitness plans that promise equally dramatic results. I, like so many others I know today, live a mostly sedentary life due to the nature of my job. And the busyness of life leaves most of us little time to get up and work out after the day is done. It's a relief to see how Joey sees that, acknowledges the challenges, and spells out how even the simplest changes in our habits (as doable as standing more or changing our water temperature in the shower!) can have an enormous impact on our overall health. It turns out that the little things really *do* matter, and that's a huge comfort to hear from someone as experienced and knowledgeable as Joey.

What's great about Joey, other than his ability to break down the language of fitness and health into bite-sized pieces, is his realness and vulnerability. It's what draws people to him—myself included—and it makes him stand out from all the other industry voices vying for our attention. His methods, tips, and tricks aren't just about eating better and getting more exercise; he's focused on your entire well-being—your mental and emotional health included. He's been honest with both me and his audience about his personal struggles with mental health and having "off" days, and invites us to accept those days as normal, not something to be ignored, and definitely not something to be punished.

This isn't a book that demands your all, every hour of every day. It's a book that encourages you to make small changes that build into big, real results, written by someone trustworthy and determined to make sure others don't fall into the same fitness traps and myths with which he's so familiar.

The work Joey is doing is powerful stuff and I'm proud to call him my friend. I appreciate him immensely for what he's been up to and for the ways he's changing the conversation around fitness, busting harmful myths, and spurring people on to start and maintain realistic, yet life-changing, regimens. He's a good man doing good work, and I hope you'll join him and so many others on a fitness journey fueled by truth and accessibility to all—and requiring only the minimum effort for maximum results!

—Dr. Will Cole
New York Times bestselling author of *Intuitive Fasting*

Preface

I'm sorry. I truly am.

Now, this may be a strange way to start a book, but I am truly sorry for all of the confusion and hurt I have caused you. I made you feel that you needed to do more and more to achieve your goals. I made you feel unworthy and worthless. I made you feel as if no matter what changes you made, there would be something new around the corner.

The *I* that I'm referring to is me and the entire fitness, health, and diet industries. We have come to think—and tell you—that you need to crush it every single day. We've made you believe that you should wake up every day thinking today is going to be amazing. We've treated you as if you don't have—or are entitled to—normal human emotions. We are the ones who told you that everything will be better when, dammit, sometimes things won't get better for a long time.

One of the single most important truths that we have never told you is that it is okay not to be okay. It is okay to have bad days. It is okay not to give every workout your all. It is okay if the scale moves in the wrong direction. It is even okay to eat carbs!

For a long time, I was one of those guys who thought I had to do more, more, more to keep fit and to keep up with the fitness industry. I've been interested in sports and exercise for as long as I can remember—biking, running, and playing team sports as a kid. For a long time it seemed I had to keep trying to level up my practice, even when it didn't actually need to be leveled up, just for the sake of doing more, being better, and getting stronger. I was five years old when I started playing soccer and hockey, and I played hockey through college. I knew that I wasn't good enough to make a lot of money playing hockey (and yes, these teeth are real), but by then I had found this new love for lifting weights. So I threw my energy into that. From there, it was a quick path to getting certified as a personal trainer, grabbing all my stuff, and driving my yellow Mustang (yes, it was yellow) to Chicago to start my career in the fitness world.

As the years went by, I went from the headstrong, energetic guy who had a passion for lifting weights and working out to realizing I needed to educate myself more to understand the reasons behind what I was doing. I went from being the guy in college who studied just enough to keep my grades up to play hockey to realizing what I really loved was learning the true science of health and fitness. The more I learned, the more I started questioning the way the majority of the fitness industry was approaching how we should look at ourselves and treat ourselves. But it still took me a long time to get out of the "more is more" and "bigger is better" mindset that dominates the fitness world I loved and to realize that maybe we are actually doing too much! As a lifelong athlete, I might be able to push myself and keep up with the standard of increasingly strenuous, lengthy workouts. But this approach was not working for many of my clients. Switching my mindset from a goal of constant escalation to more efficient and effective practices that actually get the best results changed my life and the lives of my clients.

And that's why we're here.

I'm writing this book for you, for me, and for anyone who is fed up with having to live their life at full throttle. Here's the thing about hitting the gas and accelerating. You will get to your destination, but so will the person using cruise control. Some people have that all-out effort all of the time, but most people don't.

We are human. That means we are flawed. We make mistakes. And we have insecurities. All of our humanness plays a major role in our health journey, and for too long, the fitness industry has ignored that. Well, no more. Whether your goal is to drop some weight, feel more confident in your body, or simply feel more inspired and energized, you have to address your entire self. That includes all those pesky insecurities and negative thought patterns that serve as nothing but roadblocks on your journey.

My hope is that you put some of my advice—even if it's just one thing—into action. My hope is that you choose to truly show up for yourself. But if today is not that day, that's okay. There's always tomorrow.

The fitness and nutrition industries are often looked at as superficial; they're all about how you look on the outside. And maybe for some people, this is most important. But I believe achieving a happy and healthy life is not about how you train or what you eat. It's about how you *feel*. It's about holistic health. And that's my intention for this book—to address all the aspects of you, and, more importantly, to allow you to be *you*.

Let this book be a guide, not an instruction manual. As you read it, pay attention to how you feel. Notice your limiting beliefs and try not to let them get the best of you. Information is rarely black-and-white—that's as much true for health and wellness as it is for anything else. So I give you permission to find your gray.

When it comes to health, nutrition, and fitness, there's a lot of data out there, and it can get overwhelming and confusing. Those who aren't professional athletes or scientists studying the human body don't really need all that information. That's why I'm so excited to share *The Minimum Method* with you—it takes all the confusing, all-over-the-place data on fitness and nutrition and distills it into simple, actionable, digestible information that can help you achieve lasting change.

Life is a journey, and it can often feel as if we are just along for the ride, as if we are just living the story. But in reality we are writing it. It's never too late to add another chapter to your story. As you read this book, always keep in mind that you are the author of your story. You are in charge of your life. It is yours and yours alone. So go ahead and grab that metaphorical pen because we have a lot of pages to write.

Introduction

The Minimum Method & You

Let's make a deal.

Each time I meet a new client, whether they are a celebrity training for a movie role or a new mom wanting to lose her baby weight, we start with the same conversation. I lay all my cards on the table—from what I can promise them to what I expect from them—and they have to agree with how we are going to approach reaching their health goals before we move forward.

In any client-trainer relationship, both people must do their parts to see results. As trainers, we must be dedicated to both teaching and learning—coaching our clients on exercise and nutrition while staying on top of the latest science and research in the field.

Think about it: how often do we as a society ever really *know* something? We knew the earth was flat until we learned it wasn't. We knew the atom was the smallest particle in the universe until we split it. Smoking first hit the scene as a healthy alternative to dessert, and now look what we know about it! How we trained people twenty years ago is not the same as how we train them today. Research changes and our thinking evolves. The point is we must be willing to learn, which means accepting when we are wrong or misinformed.

It drives me crazy when someone can't admit they were wrong or when information is lacking validity. We can only become better at what we do when we take a step back to assess what is working and what is not working. I'm always willing to learn new ways to become more efficient at what I do and helping my clients achieve their goals. The best thing I can hear from a client is that they don't need me anymore.

As fitness professionals continue to learn more about the human body and how it interacts with food and exercise, we learn new and better ways to help our clients. These ways require discipline and an open mind willing to let go of old beliefs and learn new ways of thinking and approaching our craft. And it's no coincidence that those are the exact characteristics we need from clients to be successful.

You need to be willing to replace old habits and thoughts with ones that better serve you. And you need to be disciplined. I can't come into your house and make you put away the cookie dough at 1 AM, tell you to go to bed earlier, or convince you to take more moments for yourself instead of always giving to others.

That's the deal we need to make at this very moment. It took a lot of discipline and a lot of research for me to write this book. Now it's on you to have an open mind while reading it, a willingness to make changes, and the willpower to take action.

So here are all my cards . . .

My goal with *The Minimum Method* is to teach you the bare essentials to improve your health. And, yes, I do mean the absolute bare minimum that is required for you to take your body to the next level, whether that means getting off the couch and just starting to exercise, finally losing those last couple of inches to hit your longtime body fat percentage goal, optimizing your sleep, or anything in between. No matter where you are on your fitness journey, this book can help you.

But notice that I said *can* help you, not *will* help you. That's an important distinction. I'm going to arm you with all the knowledge you need to reach your goals, but knowledge can only take you so far. It's up to you to do the work. I'm sorry, but there's just no way around that. This isn't a book that you can simply read and magically get results. We are a product of our effort—or lack thereof. This book will give you the path, but you have to walk it. This is not a book for people looking for shortcuts.

The Minimum Method will go back to basics, focusing on where all great journeys start: the beginning. If you are someone who is already fit, this book will teach you how to optimize your practice and perhaps get a little more time back in your day. You might even start getting better results by spending less time pumping iron and more time on your breathwork—don't look at me like that, it's true.

Ultimately, here is my promise to you: every piece of advice in this book will contribute to an actual result. I'm not going to waste your time making you sweat just for the sake of sweating, and I'm not going to ask you to live by superfluous standards that aren't actually rooted in research.

Now, what do you promise me? Come on, say it out loud!

Okay, cool—we have a deal.

LESS REALLY CAN BE MORE

Am I really going to tell you to give the minimum effort? Yes, that's for real. But, as I've said, that comes with a caveat—you still have to do the work. You have to start down the path. I will lay it out for you, but you have to take each step. And despite my best efforts, *minimum* does not always mean "easy." I've done my best to make sure that every step is as easy as possible, but any book or program that makes a blanket promise of being so easy is either lying to you or not actually doing anything for you.

In the pages that follow, we're going to establish some clear and realistic goals. And remember, this is not about trying to lose 10 pounds in ten days with some crazy detox method. Do you own one of those books? If you do, my guess is you started to read it and didn't get through it because you quickly realized—and you were right—that it was insane. If you did manage to get through it and follow the program, how'd it go? I'm assuming you weren't able to keep the weight off, or you wouldn't have picked up this book.

I'm fed up with the onslaught of "health" books that promote extreme measures to achieve a goal. They do nothing but stress people out and set them up for failure instead of long-term success. The Minimum Method is as much a mindset shift as it is a practical program. I want you to know that you can lose weight, build muscle, eat well, and feel smarter and happier in your own body without going full beast mode. You can have a body that you're proud to show off at the beach without becoming a biohacking nerd (I did that for you—no worries!) or a peak performer. I'll show you how doing simple little things can create big changes.

I'm going to be honest—changing your mindset is easier said than done. We've all spent too much time swimming in the waters of "give it your all" and "no pain, no gain" and "how to get the perfect shredded body in twenty-eight days" to be able to just accept that there can actually be benefits to giving minimal effort. So before we dive into the minimum tools for optimizing your thinking, breathing, eating, sleeping, exercising, and recovering, I'll demonstrate why minimum effort can actually be more effective than maximum effort when it comes to physical results, and why our culture of "pushing it to the limit" is actually hurting us and keeping us from achieving our goals.

Take sleep, for example. In addition to being a personal trainer, I am a certified sleep science coach. We're often told that we absolutely need eight hours of sleep every night to be healthy. The Minimum Method asks, what about your sleep quality? In chapter two, I'm going to teach you about sleep hygiene and good sleep vs. more sleep. After you've practiced positive sleep hygiene and are actually getting good sleep, you can start to figure out how much sleep you need to wake up feeling refreshed and energized before your alarm goes off. Sure, some people need a solid nine hours even if their sleep hygiene is perfect, but many people need as few as six hours of *good* sleep to be happy, healthy, and ready for the day. This is how we apply the Minimum Method to sleep.

Here's another example: do you need to attend yoga classes for several hours each week to become more flexible? I certainly won't stop you if that's something you want to do, but the answer is no, you don't need to do that. You can increase your flexibility in just five minutes, twice a day. You may not have the time or budget for a yoga membership, but I know you can pull yourself away from your desk/couch/computer for a whopping ten minutes a day. These quick five-minute sessions have the benefit of reducing stress, relieving soreness and tightness in your muscles and joints, and even boosting your metabolism and increasing fat burning. Who wouldn't want that?

Now let's talk about the minimum for weight loss, which is always a popular topic. Why do you think so many diets have been sold with the promise of no exercise? Well—to be blunt—because a lot of people are lazy and don't want to exercise. But as you'll see in later chapters, you shouldn't be exercising just because you want to lose weight. Physical activity benefits your brain function, sleep quality, and so much more. But with the Minimum Method, you don't need to be at the gym every day to gain those benefits. Many are unlocked by something as simple as one or two ten-minute walks per day.

Since weight loss is a goal for so many people picking up this book, let's talk about an important fact of weight loss that is so often glossed over in other plans and programs—weight loss is not linear! The Minimum Method will teach you how to play the long game and how to find immediate indicators of your progress beyond the scale so you can feel the satisfaction of progress. The goal here is simple—you want your weight to keep trending down over time. That means that sometimes the scale will go up, other times it will go down, sometimes it will stay the same, and all of that is okay! We just want your weight loss to be trending in the right direction over time. I'll teach you how to properly track your weight loss by using a graph. This is the most effective, sustainable strategy for weight loss. Oh, and you get to keep your sanity as well.

One of the biggest benefits of the Minimum Method is that it is designed to fit into your day. Odds are that you are not a highly paid actor whose only job over the next few months is to get fit in preparation for a role with personal trainers and nutritionists on call to make sure that happens. It's more likely that your job demands that you sit at a desk for the majority of the day. Maybe your office keeps cookies in the break room for when you do get up. You might have kids, dogs, parents, or someone else who relies on you so it's impossible for you to always put yourself first. And all of this is okay, too! You're living a normal human life. What is the point of a health and fitness plan if it can't fit into a normal human life? Why design a program for the peak when there are still so many people trying to make it up the hill?

KNOW YOUR STARTING LINE

I'm not going to sit here and pretend that everyone is at the same place in their health and wellness journey. You all have different pasts, different presents, and different desired futures. Any fitness or nutrition program that doesn't take this into account is missing the mark. Everyone's body and mind are unique, which means there isn't—and can never be—a one-size-fits-all program to help everyone achieve their goals. So in the absence of being able to meet with each of you individually, here's how we're going to address this important (yet overlooked) element of any fitness book.

First, we need to get a clear picture of your past habits and lifestyle. This will inform where you need to start and also help set realistic expectations. The time it takes to change is heavily influenced by how long you've been doing what you've been doing. For example, let's look at two different people—Person 1 and Person 2. Let's pretend both are the same gender, have the same general body type, and are the same height, weight, and body mass index (BMI). (As you will find out in later chapters, BMI is kind of BS, but we'll use it for this analogy.) They're as close to physically identical as you can get. There is just a major lifestyle difference: Person 1 has been inactive and eating poorly for the past ten years, and Person 2 used to be more fit but gained unwanted weight in 2020 (as many people did due to the Covid-19 pandemic). It's incorrect to assume that because they're seemingly starting at the same place, their journey will look the same. Because that's the thing—they're not starting at the same place.

Think of it like walking up a hill. Person 2 was already halfway up the hill and then stopped and sat down. Person 1 has been chillin' at the base of the hill for a decade. When they both decide to stand up and walk, their journey to the top of the hill will be different in every way. Person 2's legs are already used to walking uphill while Person 1 may need to ease into the hike. Person 2 will see more elevation progress with every step while Person 1 will cover more distance at first because the ground is flatter at the base of the hill.

You see, there are so many factors that determine what kind of shape you are in now, your ability to lose fat or gain muscle, how you handle sugar, how you process food, and so much more. We all have different metabolisms, genetic factors, limb lengths, past injuries, and the list goes on and on. It doesn't make sense to compare or compete with others. *Average* doesn't really exist. There is only your accumulation of your own life experiences. Self-assessment is the only meaningful data. Our bodies change over the years and adapt to the current stimuli we are placing on them. It's great that you played high school football thirty years ago, but your body is much different now. You have accumulated a lot of miles, and your system needs to be checked and tuned up regularly. If only we could trade in our brains and bodies for newer models every couple of years!

So we need to check in on your system and find out where on the hill you're starting. Honestly answer the following questions:

- How many hours of sleep have you been getting? Do you wake up feeling rested?
- How stressed do you feel?
- How often do you do something active?
- How much water do you drink on a daily basis?
- How much processed food do you eat?

Think about your answers for this current chapter of your life, and also for your past chapters. What are your answers for your life three months ago? A year ago? Ten years ago? All of this affects where you are now.

> For a worksheet to help you complete this exercise, go to joeythurman.com/homework.

Why did I have you answer those questions? If I were to only look at what you did over the past week, it may look perfect to you and to me. But that isn't the overall picture, right? Maybe you have been incredibly stressed this year and felt extra tired and put on weight. Maybe ten years ago you didn't have as many responsibilities or children and slept better. Your twenty-four hours today may look different than they did years ago. It really ticks me off when I hear someone say that we all have the same twenty-four hours in a day. Um, no, we don't! The single mom working two jobs has much less time for herself than someone who has more help. Be aware of your time and assess where you can fit you in! We have to know where you have been so we can determine where you can start right now. I will say this over and over again—what you do today affects your tomorrow, and what you do tomorrow keeps you on your path.

Now it's time for an important step—acceptance. Accept where you are right now and where you have been at every stage of your life. You can't change the past, it's already happened. You can't even change the present because it's already here. All we can ever change is the future, and—ironically—we do that in the present. Right now is the moment we start to change your life. And you have to start by accepting where you are and where you've been. Holding on to regret or *I wish I would have*s or *I knew I shouldn't*s will only hinder your progress. Every moment is an opportunity to start clean, and that's what you need to do right now. As for everything that has led to this moment, let . . . it . . . all . . . go. From here on, we will only look forward.

Actually, that's a lie. You will sometimes need to come back to this moment and maybe even think about your past—but for one reason and one reason only:

to remember and celebrate progress. As you move forward, there will be times when you get discouraged and times when you don't feel like you're getting anywhere. That's when you look back at the answers to the above questions to remind yourself of how far you've come. How much stronger do you feel? How much more energy do you have? How much better are you eating and sleeping?

The road ahead won't always be easy, so right now I want you to give yourself permission to suck. I'm about to give you a ton of information and a lot of it will probably be new to you and sometimes tough. But no one picks up an instrument they've never played and is immediately a master at it. So don't expect yourself to be. Instead, embrace the suck.

THERE'S MORE THAN ONE WAY TO READ THIS BOOK

Each chapter in this book will give you the tools to do the minimum and get the maximum out of different aspects of life. I'm talking about sleep, exercise, brain habits for mental efficiency, breathwork to combat stress, nutrition to make you look and feel better, and more. As a whole, this book gives you the opportunity and know-how to improve every part of your life. But that doesn't mean you have to read the book in its entirety to get anything out of it. You can choose to only read the chapters that interest you or even read them out of order if you'd like. Each chapter is designed to stand on its own, and there's a reason for that. Change in any form can be overwhelming. I don't want you to think you have to read this book from cover to cover to get any benefits from it. I fully recognize that could be overwhelming.

Change is only accomplished one step at a time. Within each chapter are several steps you can take to change your life. Take each step as you are ready for it. And when you're ready for more, come back to the book and read another chapter. The point is to get better a little bit at a time. You don't have to overhaul your entire life in a matter of weeks. For most people, that isn't sustainable. At the end of the day, I want you to achieve lasting change.

And here's something most fitness experts won't tell you—some days you will not be better. Some days you will be worse, and some days you will be the same. Just as weight loss isn't linear, neither is change. Some days you'll have good moments and some days you'll have bad moments. It's what you do with those days and moments that matter to keep you trending toward your health goals.

My hope is that you implement these tools one by one so you can reach your maximum results. Remember, we're not falling into the fitness myth that more is always better. Most of us are searching for the starting line, not the finish line. You may be struggling to get off the couch, and that is okay! We're not striving for maximum effort. Our goal is efficiency. The least effort for the most gain.

1

YOU MUST UNLEARN TO LEARN

LIAR, LIAR: THE INDUSTRY'S PANTS ARE ON FIRE

We are constantly bombarded with so many images and messages—and yes, including books and fitness programs like this one—telling us what we're supposed to look like and how we're supposed to get there. I'm going to let you in on a little secret: most of it is BS. And worse, it's BS that's after your wallet.

Pick up any magazine or turn on any blockbuster movie and you'll likely see a popular celebrity in peak physical condition. It's often images like this that inspire people to start working out. How can you not feel the urge to start working out while looking at living proof that perfection is possible? That proof gets you all motivated, and before you know it, you're going down a rabbit hole, searching for celebrity trainer workout videos. And as we all know, there's no shortage of fitness and nutrition programs out there. This is by design.

For years, the health industry has created and capitalized on the latest and greatest workouts and diets. In 1975, tons of people went on a cookie diet. No, I'm not exaggerating. People bought these cookies that supposedly had a special hunger-controlling formula and ate them throughout the day to curb their appetite. Then, in the 1980s, everyone was stocking up on cabbage for the cabbage soup diet. People literally ate nothing but cabbage soup for a week. With both diets, people may have lost some weight initially but it didn't stay off, and it wasn't the weight they wanted to lose.

Here's the thing. If you've been eating too much for a long time, any sort of calorie deprivation will most likely lead to some sort of weight loss. But more often than not, you're losing muscle or water weight—not fat—and the weight will return before you can even take the tags off your new smaller-size pair of pants. Simply put, any kind of quick fix diet will not be effective or sustainable. You may temporarily lose some weight, but you'll feel like crap doing it and feel even worse when the weight returns.

Fad diets and workouts all have the same goal in mind: get our attention, take our dollars, and beat the competition. It's a massive industry. In 2019, the weight loss market was worth $72 billion![1] But despite the best intentions of many people within that market, it's still an industry designed to make money, whether you actually get healthy or not.

Still, with all those exercises and meal plans going around, you'd think we'd be an extremely healthy nation. That is sadly not the case. Instead, obesity rates continue to rise. In 2019, the obesity rate in the United States was 39.6 percent. Only one year later, it jumped up to 42 percent.[2] That is more than 139 million friends, neighbors, family members, and coworkers who struggle with obesity.

Obesity itself isn't the issue. The issue is the repercussions of obesity. An obese person is at higher risk of contracting all causes of death, heart disease, stroke, several types of cancer, gallbladder disease, depression, anxiety, and the list goes on.[3] So, what do we do with this information? How do we change the situation?

Diet culture certainly isn't the answer. It's arguably caused more pain and suffering for people than it has actually helped because it's not our size that matters, but how we feel. Do you wake up feeling refreshed or must you pry yourself out of bed? Do you feel energized throughout the day or does the post-lunch lull get you down? Do you easily move about pain-free, or do you struggle to get out of the car or up from a chair? Are you able to get down on the floor to play with your dog, children, or grandchildren? Simply put, are you able to do the activities in life that you want to do (and have to do) and feel good while doing them?

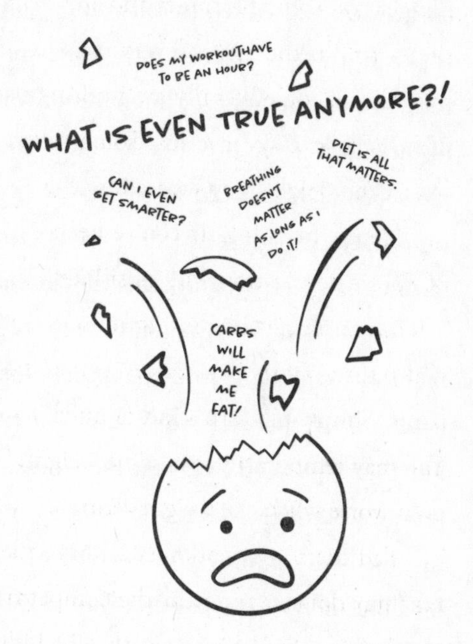

The sad truth is that most people today don't feel good. Even sadder, most people don't know what it's like to feel good because they've felt lousy for so long it's become their norm. I'm on a mission to change that. Everyone deserves to feel good, and everyone has the ability to feel good. It starts by changing the narrative. I want you to wrap your head around this statement: instead of constantly chasing weight loss to get healthy, what if you get healthy and then lose weight?

It's time to set the record straight. Let's debunk some of the most common myths about fitness.

Myth #1: Perfection Is the Goal

This is one of the biggest myths in fitness: that we can (and, by that implication, should) achieve and sustain the perfect body and walk around with low single-digit body fat numbers—which isn't even healthy! We need some fat on our bodies to maintain bodily functions, for our brains to work effectively, and, if you are a woman, to have a regular menstrual cycle.

As someone who has helped many celebrities reach what you probably think of as physical perfection, I'll let you in on a little secret: they do not look like that most of the time! What you see is nothing more than a snapshot that's created, lit, and edited to sell you on something. Getting their bodies in shape is part of these celebrities' jobs. Someone like me is hired to prepare them for a role, awards ceremony, or photo shoot, and I'm paid to dial in every single aspect of their lives, from their habits and workouts to their sleep, nutrition, and supplements. Here's a little secret—sometimes I even put them in contact with the right doctors to prescribe the perfect potion, usually a mix of specific peptides, testosterone therapy, and other not-so-mainstream supplements.

Their physique is the only aspect of life these celebrities are focused on for months. It's all done to prepare them for that perfect moment in time, whether it be a photo shoot or movie role. The rest of the year they don't look anything like that. But people all over the world still hang those pictures on mirrors and refrigerators as a visual reminder of their goals. That one picture-perfect moment in time lives on forever in people's minds as an example of what they want to look like, or, worse, what they should look like. Let me tell you this—you cannot look like anyone else and no one can look like you (unless you are an identical twin). We all have different bodies, lives, metabolisms, limb lengths, medications we were prescribed as kids that messed up our microbiomes, stressors, endocrine fluctuations . . . need I go on?

Does this mean you can't lose weight and look great in pants several sizes smaller than the ones you're wearing right now? Nope, you can absolutely do that! Does it mean that you can't become lean and muscular or that abs are totally out of the question? Of course not! What we're talking about here is reasonable goal setting so you're not comparing yourself to a body you saw in a magazine and feeling disappointed with anything short of that very specific (and again, temporary at best) image. That type of disappointment is discouraging and can lead you to give up before you have a chance to make real progress.

So how do you set realistic expectations of yourself so you don't get discouraged? Well, if I've said it once, I've said it a million times—you can only look like you! Your goals need to reflect that.

There are, in fact, different body types that are in some part determined by bone structure. These include, for example, leg and torso length, hip width, and spine curvature. We also tend to store fat differently, which is somewhat determined by genetics. Some people store more fat in their midsection, whereas others carry it more in their thighs or arms. Hormones also play a role—stress-induced cortisol, estrogen, and progesterone can all affect fat distribution.

That being said, claiming to be big-boned is not necessarily a valid statement. It is true that some people have a larger frame, but most of our weight comes from soft tissue (fat, muscle, and organs), not from bones. Let's go ahead and calculate body frame size for fun.

Your body frame size is based on height and wrist circumference. So use a tape measure to measure your wrist, then use these guidelines[4] to determine your frame size:

	Women's Frame Size		
Height	**Small**	**Medium**	**Large**
Under 5′2″	Wrist size is less than 5.50″	Wrist size is 5.50″ to 5.75″	Wrist size is more than 5.75″
5′2″ to 5′5″	Wrist size is less than 6.00″	Wrist size is 6.00″ to 6.25″	Wrist size is more than 6.25″
5′5″ and up	Wrist size is less than 6.25″	Wrist size is 6.25″ to 6.50″	Wrist size is more than 6.50″

	Men's Frame Size		
Height	**Small**	**Medium**	**Large**
5'5" and up	Wrist size is 5.50" to 6.50"	Wrist size is 6.50" to 7.50"	Wrist size is more than 7.50"

So when setting goals and expectations, you need to take into account everything mentioned above. Some of it you can proactively manage, like your stress response and cortisol levels. And some of it you can't, like where you store fat. A weight loss journey needs to be equal parts work and body acceptance.

Myth #2: Your Workout Should Last an Hour

When you think about it, this is absurd. Who came up with the idea that to achieve results, workouts had to be a specific length of time? I'm sure right now you're thinking back to a recent study you read that recommended how much physical activity we all should be getting. I'm not saying those studies are wrong, but I'm also not saying they're right.

The length of a workout isn't what determines how efficient or effective it is. We've all seen the guy at the gym who spends an hour on the bench press because he's checking his social media (or himself in the mirror!) after every set. Has he gotten a better workout than the person who knocks their sets out in twenty minutes?

We need to get past this notion that longer equals better. There is nothing wrong with an hour-long safe workout. But, as I will discuss later in the book, there are also benefits to shorter workouts throughout the day. The point is to remove whatever mental programming you have about how long your workout *should* be. There's just no one-size-fits-all answer so be wary of any recommendation you read about.

For example, a study in the *Journal of the American Medical Association* showed that middle-aged women who exercised an hour a day were better able to maintain their weight over thirteen years than women who didn't. At first glance, the takeaway recommendation from this study is to exercise an hour a day. But dig deeper into the study and you'll learn that the scientists didn't consider an hour to be a straight measurement of time. Instead, they looked at metabolic equivalent (MET) hours. MET hours take into account the amount of energy a body uses, with the baseline being how much energy—or calories—the body burns at rest (also known as the resting metabolic rate while awake). When you're just chilling on your couch for an hour, your body is still burning calories to function. Let's call that one MET. Spend that same hour on a walk, and you're burning calories equivalent to about three METs. Use that hour to go for a run, and you're using upward of ten METs. You see my point—the more intense the activity, the higher the METs.

This changes the way you look at the recommendation to work out for an hour, right? Sure, you can go on a walk for an hour each day, or you can do a High-Intensity Interval Training (HIIT) workout for twenty minutes. But that doesn't mean every workout needs to be HIIT and totally kick your ass. We are constantly being told that we need to work out as hard as we can and push ourselves to the limits. Words like *grinding* and phrases like *no pain, no gain* come to mind. Here's another little secret—that's just a bunch of motivational speaker BS.

Yes, some of your workouts should challenge you both physically and mentally. But there's a difference between being challenged and being stupid. Working out to the point where you can barely move or you're pushing through pain does nothing more than make you more prone to injury. We need to push our bodies just past the point of what they are used to in order to create a beneficial response.

The bottom line is to stop getting hung up on studies, recommendations, and fitness influencer pep talks, and instead find a routine that works for you. We'll discuss this more in chapter eight.

There is a balance with getting in the proper amount of resistance training, cardio, and making sure your body has the proper amount of time to recover. Too much too fast can do more harm than good, it's all about listening to your body and following the science. I'll give you the down and dirty on all of that in chapter six.

Myth #3: I Must Do Cardio

If you truly want to change the shape of your body, you need to chill out on the cardio. I realize reading that may make some of you angry, but I'm not here to coddle you. I'm here to tell you the truth and give you tools so you can decide how you want to control your life. There's a reason so many people gravitate toward that useless elliptical machine or walk on a treadmill in the gym—because it's easy! It requires zero thought or know-how. I'm not saying cardio isn't good for you or instructing you not to do it at all. As you will read later in this book, I will give you specific cardio and movement recommendations. The point I want to make is that there is a time and place for cardio.

In some cases, a lot of cardio will do more harm than good. Extended bouts of cardio create a stress response in your body. This stress increases cortisol levels and up-regulates the storage of fat, especially if we don't do what's required to recover after exercise or get chronic cortisol elevations down during the day. A lot of acute stressors are good, even inflammation can be good at times, but we don't want chronically elevated levels. Too much cardio tells the body that a stressful event is happening, and it needs to switch from burning fat to storing it and use muscle tissue for energy instead.

So why are we constantly being sold on cardio as the best way to burn the calories needed to reach our fitness goals? I'll give you a little hint: currently, over sixty million people own treadmills, and in-home bikes are all the rage (how many times have you heard someone mention Peloton in the last few months?). Do you think those companies care about consumers understanding the truth about cardio? No way—they're too busy counting their money.

Cardio can help you burn calories, but the truth of the matter is it only burns calories (for the most part) during the cardio session itself. If someone were to ask me what they should do if they have only an hour a week to work out, my answer would be resistance training. If they have only two hours, my answer would be the same. Then maybe after that, we would have a talk about adding cardio. With other forms of exercise—like weight training and interval training—the metabolic rate stays elevated after the workout is finished, which means the body keeps burning calories and fat after the workout.

Myth #4: Weight Training Will Make You Bulky

This one might be my favorite because I hear it so often from my female clients. Ladies, once and for all—lifting weights will not make you big or bulky. And trust me, you want to put on some muscle. Why? Well here are just a few of the benefits:

- Muscle burns more calories than fat.
- Muscle improves insulin sensitivity and lowers the risk for prediabetes.[5]
- Muscle helps your other workouts be more efficient.
- Muscle protects your joints.
- Muscle improves your balance and coordination.

Okay, so now that you're pro-muscle, let's talk more about it. Here's a fact—all muscle is lean. There is no difference between lean muscle tissue and bulky muscle tissue. What makes a person look lean or bulky isn't the amount of muscle they have; it's the amount of fat they're carrying on top of the muscle. That's why when we focus on building muscle mass, we're aiming to do so without also gaining fat. Bulking, on the other hand, involves intentionally eating more calories than your body needs in an effort to put on mass that will ultimately consist of both muscle and fat.

Weight training alone will not make you bulky. Weight training and overeating might, which is why it's important that we always approach weight loss and health goals from a holistic approach.

Myth #5: It's All About Diet and Exercise

If it were that simple, this book would only have two chapters: one on diet and the other on exercise. Diet and exercise may get the majority of airtime in the health and fitness space, but reaching your health potential is about so much more. If I had to simplify, I would say you need sleep, diet, and exercise to reach your potential. For most of you reading this book, getting quality sleep is hands down the absolute first step you should take. Without quality sleep, all the diets and exercise programs in the world don't stand a chance. We'll do a deep dive into sleep in chapter two.

All in all, the body is a system and needs to be treated that way. If your system has been put through the ringer over the past couple of years, you need to take that into consideration when creating a workout protocol. That's why you're going to start by looking at the past and what you've been doing for the last decade or so. Then you will tackle the present—not just what should be changed, but what can be changed. This goes back to realistic expectations and goal setting.

SO WHAT'S THE TRUTH?

The fitness industry in general is getting it wrong. And for some reason, even though we've all been burned by it in some form or another, we keep falling into the next fad or trap. We need to stop listening to "research" with ulterior motives and stop letting money-hungry companies direct what we do with our bodies. They don't care about us. They care about the bottom line. I'm asking you to take a step back and look at all the demands and expectations you're placing on yourself, what advice you've been taking too seriously, and who you've been comparing yourself to. Then do the hard work of being honest about what it's doing to you.

You'll be happier and healthier doing the Minimum Method. You won't be settling for less when it comes to results; you'll be changing your mindset. The fact is that more isn't always better or more effective. You don't need more equipment, more weight, more time, more reps, or more cardio. Achieving your best body is about what's right for you, and that changes over time. You may need to level up and add more to your workout sometimes, scale back at other times, and have a full understanding of why you are doing either. This is the end of doing more for the sake of more, but fair warning: I'm not giving you a pass to do less than the minimum either.

The Minimum Method is a health plan for maximizing efficiency and efficacy, but it's not about effortlessness. Change is never easy. The Minimum Method will challenge both your body and your mind. Yes, getting your goal physique is just as much about your mind as it is about your body. In fact, it all starts with your mind.

YOUR MIND MATTERS

I told you we were going to go back to the beginning, and I meant that. Now imagine yourself as a baby. Or if you have children, go back to the day they were born. I'm not a religious person, but the closest I've ever been to a perfect being is my son, Frederic, when I was watching his birth. After children are born, they are full of light. They don't know hate or judgment or even fear. They are the epitome of innocence and add a magical essence to this world. And every experience to them is just that—magical—because it's brand new. And then what happens? Well, life happens.

We all came into this world as clean slates—no concept of how relationships should be, what we should believe, how we should act, what we should or shouldn't eat, how often we should be active, or what our bodies should look like. We didn't have bad habits or good habits. We were instinctual—we cried when we were uncomfortable and slept when we were tired.

As clean slates, we were also like big sponges, continuously taking in and learning from the world around us. We watched people and listened to them. We noticed how they interacted with each other and the decisions they made. We started asking why every chance we could. More so than they probably realized, our parents, teachers, siblings, grandparents—everyone and anyone in our life—molded and shaped us. All that input started to form our subconscious beliefs and patterns. We began to learn *shoulds* and *shouldn'ts,* and we picked up habits good and bad.

By the time we reached adulthood, we'd accumulated years and years of that stuff, and it gained a major stronghold on how we now perceive ourselves and life in general. There are the surface-level thoughts we're aware of like *my arms are fat*, and the deep-rooted stuff we aren't aware of like *I don't deserve to be happy.* It's as if we've been programmed.

I know the thought of being programmed can be unsettling, but stay with me. We've all been programmed by the environment we grew up in and the experiences we've had within that environment. In his book *The Biology of Belief,* Dr. Bruce Lipton shares that most of our subconscious is formed in the early years of our life. Our subconscious is the program that's always running in the background. We aren't even aware of it most of the time. We can thank our subconscious for allowing us to walk and breathe without thinking about it. But our subconscious is also responsible for other reactions we have without thinking, like getting frustrated in traffic, snapping at our significant other, or grabbing that cookie when we are sad. These behaviors happen so fast that they often feel automatic, as if we don't have a choice. But here's some life-changing news—we always have a choice.

Changing our subconscious patterns starts with awareness. We have to become aware of our thought cycles to change them. You can start by becoming aware after the fact. After an argument or an upsetting event, take a minute to think back and identify your thought cycle. How did you react to certain things that were said or done? How did you feel? What did you decide to do? Replaying events as conversations in your mind and analyzing them is an effective way to start identifying your patterns. The more you do this, the better you'll be able to see patterns as they're unfolding in real time. That's when you have the opportunity to make changes.

Identifying and understanding your patterns are not easy tasks. That's why therapy can be so useful. Sometimes it takes an outside perspective to see the full picture of how you operate. And I mean a total outside perspective—not a family member or friend. Their view of you will always be impacted by their past experiences with you.

We aren't completely run by the subconscious programming we picked up in childhood, though. We are still active participants in our life. You see, life is full of experiences and reactions. Things happen to us or around us, and we react. Stimuli and response. We usually can't control the stimuli, but we can always control the response.

How do we control our response, Joey? you may wonder. I'm glad you asked. Our response is usually dependent on how we view life. Change your viewpoint and suddenly you have more response options. You have a choice, and with choice comes the opportunity to change—the opportunity to reprogram your subconscious. This is conceptual, I know, so let's look at some concrete examples.

You're stuck in traffic and you're going to be late to a meeting. That sucks, but ultimately there's nothing you can do to change it, right? Your choice lies in your response. You can sit there stewing in anger and frustration while your blood pressure rises and your body goes into fight-or-flight mode, or you can see this as a gift of time—a chance to finally listen to that podcast you've been wanting to hear or call that friend or family member you've been meaning to catch up with.

Another example could be your partner forgetting to pick up the dry cleaning on their way home. When you look at just the facts, it's a simple mistake. But your subconscious programming may have you believing it's evidence that you're not a priority and your partner doesn't care about your needs. What you believe is ultimately your choice.

For an exercise to help you identify your subconscious programming, go to joeythurman.com/homework.

When we consciously seek out the good in ourselves, others, and the world around us—getting back to the beginning and into our baby mindset—we can stop seeing life as something that's out to get us, and instead see it for the magical place we once believed it was. Perception really is reality.

MIND OVER MATTER

You all agree now that you have choices, right? Those choices are key because they are what's creating your experience. At this point, many of your decisions may be reactionary and hidden within your subconscious programming, and that's okay. But now it's time to bring them all to light.

My son has a book called *What Should Danny Do?* by Ganit and Adir Levy. Throughout the story, Frederic gets to choose what Danny does in different situations in his life. When we turn the page based on my son's answer, we see what happens as a result of Danny's—or really Frederic's—choice. When it's a "bad" decision, Danny either gets in trouble or doesn't get what he wants.

I love this book for my son because it teaches him there are consequences for every decision he makes. Heck, it's one of Newton's laws—for every action, there is an equal and opposite reaction. But what I also love about this book is that it teaches we are forever writing our story. After Danny and Frederic make a "bad" decision, they still have a chance to make a "good" decision and change the story.

The same is true for every fitness and weight loss journey. Right now, your health and your body are the result of the sum of all the decisions you've made in life, both big and small. Unless you're superhuman, you've made some not-so-great decisions in the past, and you're likely to make more in the future. But here's the thing—that's okay! Your story isn't over. Every single moment is a chance to make a decision that helps get you back on track. Here's the kicker, though—you can't course correct without awareness.

Let's go back to Frederic's book. In your own life, you're Danny, obviously. You're the one actually going through your life and living it. But there's also this kid—a child like my son—making your decisions for you. Think of that kid as a personification of all your subconscious programming. It's fitting because our subconscious tends to act like a child a lot of the time—often afraid and throwing tantrums when it doesn't get what it wants.

If you want to make true, lasting change in your life, you have to realize the kid is there. You have to be aware that there is a child—all your subconscious programming—who is making a lot of your decisions. And you have to be willing to look that kid in the face and say you'll take it from here. And then you have to actually take it from there. You have to make different decisions. If you never change anything, nothing will ever change. Seems obvious but reread that slowly: if you never change anything, nothing will ever change. Like Danny, you have the choice to learn from your mistakes and continuously rewrite your own story.

The days of complaining and doing nothing need to be over. The days of feeling as if you're a victim of your circumstance and don't have control of your life are gone. You are a never-ending book with endless chapters. But you have to take control of your subconscious—take the pen out of its hand—and start writing.

MIND GAMES

As we've been discussing, our minds are powerful. A mind can be a strong ally, but it can also be a major obstacle. I believe we all have two opposing voices inside of us, and we decide which voice we listen to.

One voice is discouraging and tends to be loud, overpowering, and easier to follow. Here are some examples:

- *Don't get up today.*
- *You don't need to better yourself. You have tried and failed before, why would now be any different?*
- *That's good enough.*
- *Eat that garbage food. You deserve it.*

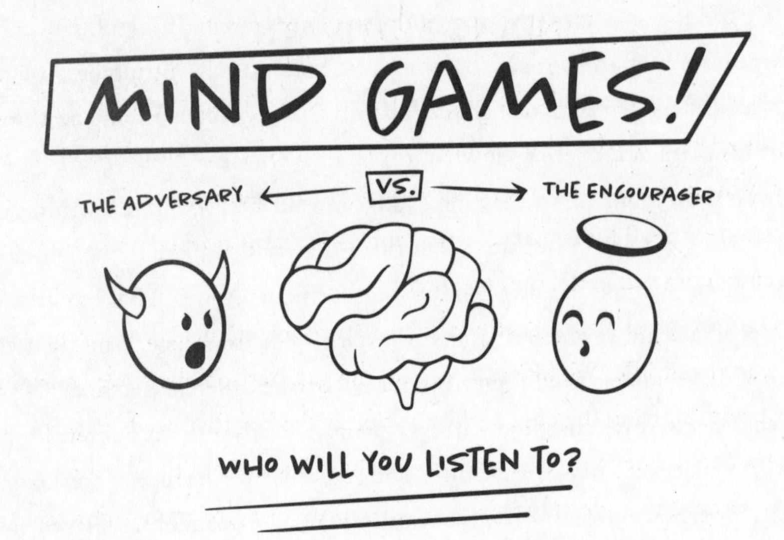

The other voice is encouraging, tends to be faint, and is often overshadowed by the loud, discouraging voice. Here are some examples:

- *You can do this. You deserve this.*
- *You can push harder.*
- *You will succeed.*
- *You will not fail this time.*
- *You will be better for you and your loved ones.*

We all have these voices in our head, and it's often easier to listen to the loudest ones. I almost listened to my loud voices today. I wanted to stay in bed. I wanted to skip my workout. I wanted to feel sorry for myself. But then I heard that quiet voice through the noise reminding me of how I would feel later for letting myself down. I'm happy to report that I let the quiet voice win! Your quiet voices won't win every time, but you will benefit from being aware of them and increasing their chances of being heard.

Let's address some quiet voice vs. loud voice battlefields in your mind that play a major role in your ability to achieve any kind of change in your life. These battlefields are motivation, progress, and failure.

FINDING MOTIVATION

You likely have some goals. Maybe your goal is weight loss related, maybe it's strength related, maybe it's mobility related, or maybe you simply want to feel better in your own skin. As long as your goal isn't some unrealistic version of "perfection," I'm all for it. Because remember—there is no true perfection; only a perception of what perfection means.

Goals are great. It's actually human nature to set them. At our core, we don't want to sit idle. We like our foot on the gas. Yet somehow, we constantly struggle with starting the engine. Motivation is the key that needs to be turned to get that engine revving and ready to put us in motion. But how do we access it? First we need to understand there are two forms of motivation—intrinsic and extrinsic—and we need both.

Intrinsic motivation is an inner need to accomplish something solely for yourself such as proving to yourself that you can learn a new language or run a Spartan Race even though you hate cardio. Okay, that was one of my intrinsic motivations.

Completing a Spartan Race was important to me because I was always the guy who played traditional team sports. The beauty of team sports is the team part—you suffer the losses and celebrate the victories with the rest of your team members. I wanted to do something on my own. I wanted to prove that I could push myself without a team relying on me or backing me up, even if that meant running four miles up a muddy mountain only stopping to crawl under barbed wire. It was really tough, but I did it.

And that's the thing about intrinsic motivation—it's usually fueled by firsts and driven by discomfort. It's hard to find intrinsic motivation doing the things you've always done. It requires you to step outside your comfort zone and push yourself to a limit you haven't reached yet. That's the motivation—to go further than you've ever been before. And the reward? Simply knowing that you can—the pride you feel in overcoming an obstacle that seemed insurmountable, or a goal that previously felt unreachable.

Extrinsic motivation, on the other hand, comes from someone else or is driven by a tangible reward, rather than those internal feelings of reward as described above. Extrinsic motivation may include wanting to look your best for someone you haven't seen in a while (hello, high school reunions) or the desire to win a competition or prize to prove your worth to others. Simply put, extrinsic motivation is driven by something outside yourself.

While extrinsic motivation is often easier to define than intrinsic motivation, that doesn't mean it's easy to hold on to. What gets in the way of our extrinsic motivation? Good old, plain excuses. And boy, do we love our excuses! I like to say that excuses are like assholes: we all have one (sorry, but it's true). As a personal trainer, I've heard every excuse imaginable. And here's what I know about excuses: they may live on the surface, but their roots run deep. It's never really about being too tired to exercise, "having" to go out for drinks, or not having time to cook a healthy meal. There's always an underlying cause (hello subconscious programming), and that's ultimately what needs to change. My job is to help you connect with both your intrinsic and extrinsic motivations, so you can overcome your underlying causes. Let's be honest, showing up to work out with me for 3 out of the 168 hours of the week isn't enough to solve all your problems and change your life. Only you can change your life. My goal is to help guide you.

CELEBRATING PROGRESS

How long did it take you to get out of shape or put on the weight you want to lose? The answer is probably years, or months at the very least. So, then, why do you think you can undo years of decisions in ten days of exercising and healthy eating? When you really think about it, it's absurd! But I also can't blame you for thinking that way. You've spent a lifetime bombarded by TV shows, advertisements, books, and influencers promising quick fixes to get your summer body in a few weeks—all of which have set you up with some seriously unrealistic expectations about when and how you're going to achieve your physical goals.

It's not just you—even people in the industry get caught up in this unhealthy mindset of "fast results." I've had friends who were producers of weight loss shows call me complaining about a lack of progress after only a few weeks. I then have to put reality into perspective—it's only been a few weeks, relax. More often than not, they're overtraining, not eating correctly, not managing their stress, and not getting enough quality sleep.

Reaching goals is great, but making progress toward goals is when life is taking place. While it's easy to think that change happens in the future (however near or distant), it actually only happens in the present. Change happens with the decision to go for a walk after dinner, the choice not to eat another cookie, and the conviction to set your alarm for the next morning's workout. Those tiny moments in life add up and either lead to progress or maintain the status quo.

A great way to hold on to your motivation is to celebrate your progress. Don't wait until you reach a goal to feel good about what you've done—celebrate each step you took along the way. So how do we define progress?

Many people consult a mirror or scale to determine progress with their health. But it's not that simple. Too often, people start feeling better and rush to a scale, excited and convinced they must have lost weight, then become overwhelmed by disappointment if the number on the scale hasn't changed yet. Allow yourself to feel that positive difference even if it isn't showing yet. Be proud of yourself for starting a new routine. Be honored that you're setting a good example for your loved ones. And be grateful that you're putting yourself first. Think about your newfound strength, your new routine, or even your new energy for life. There is always something—no matter how small—that is positive to hold on to.

Focus on moments in the present—a minimum effort that leads to a maximum reward. You're not doing tomorrow's workout right now, and you can't stick to your meal plan for the month at this very second. Those things happen when their moment comes. All you can do right now—or at any moment—is make the choice that moves you closer to your goal and be proud of yourself for doing so. Focus on the moments, celebrate progress, and trust that one day your efforts will all add up.

RETHINKING FAILURE

Let's talk about failure. Nothing kills motivation or overshadows progress more than what we perceive as failure. Let's be real here, we're all human. We are all going to have bad days and make bad decisions. Do you really think celebrities and fitness influencers eat and act perfectly every single day? No way! Remember, most of those photos you see are of them at their peak moments and don't represent how they live when someone like me isn't managing their every meal and workout in preparation for that photo. So, first, cut yourself some slack. Whether you're a professional athlete or an average Joe, you can 100 percent snap back from any kind of "failure."

We live in a culture that glorifies effortless success and "natural" ability—the gifted athlete, the drop-out genius, the talented performer who is discovered by chance rather than through years of morale-crushing auditions. People like that are the exception, not the rule. Most of us live in the real world, where goals take effort to achieve and trying something new doesn't have an immediate payoff. Anyone who has ever tried hard at something has likely failed at some point. I'm not saying that means you must fail to succeed. I'm simply saying that you are likely to fail at some point on your journey, and that's okay.

How do you deal with failure? First you need to accept that it is likely going to happen and it's actually a good thing. Without mistakes in life, how would we know what not to do? So take the word *failure* and change the meaning of it. Look at it instead as a necessity for growth. Then when you inevitably fail, you can see it for what it is—an opportunity to grow. That allows you to acknowledge it and move forward.

I want to touch on punishment before we move on. Punishment and failure are not the same, and accepting punishment is not the same as accepting failure. There are some diets and programs out there that instruct you to punish yourself for eating a food item that is not on their approved food list. Let me be perfectly clear—this kind of practice is not sustainable, does more harm than good, and pisses me off.

The punishment mindset is exactly how we got into this unhealthy situation in the first place. We think if we make one mistake in our health journey that it is the be-all and end-all. This isn't how life works and isn't how your health journey should go! I want you to be okay with not being okay. I want you to have your bad moments and your good moments. And more than anything, I want you to know that punishing yourself will lead you nowhere.

The Minimum Method isn't about doing a little, it's about understanding how little you need to do to get better! You'll make much more progress if you can take your mistakes, learn from them, let them go (this part is very important), and then move on. Failure is something you can learn from and will propel you forward, but punishment will only hold you back.

WHAT TO DO WITH ALL THOSE NEGATIVE THOUGHTS

We all have that negative voice inside our heads pointing out what's wrong with us, what's wrong with others, and what's wrong with the world. And like the discouraging voice, our negative voice can be quite loud.

We need to recognize and confront the negative thoughts that prevent us from reaching our goals. I'll go first. Here are some of the negative thoughts that I consistently battle:

- *I don't deserve success.*
- *I'm afraid of failing my son.*
- *I'm afraid of not being enough for my family.*
- *I'm constantly battling impostor syndrome.*
- *I'm scared that I won't ever find a true direction in my life.*
- *I'm terrified that my depression will get the best of me.*
- *I'm scared to death that this book will be a flop and validate all of my insecurities.*

My hope is that telling you what my insecurities are, letting down my walls and trying to break through them, will allow you to recognize and address your insecurities. Your walls are there for a reason. I never want to discount that. Your experiences up until this point in your life matter. If they left a lasting imprint, it's for a good reason. Don't try to ignore them or shove them away. You can pretend they're not there for only so long. A lot of motivational BS-ers out there tell you to quiet or silence that voice. Well, not me.

I think we can all admit that life just sucks sometimes. You need to be aware of that. Sometimes you just can't push through everything. I get that. In those times, it's a waste of energy to try to quiet or silence the negative voice. Instead, use that energy to activate your reward system. It's hard to suppress your negative thoughts but you can always add more positive thoughts. So instead of trying to have fewer negative thoughts (as so many people advise), I'm telling you to just have more positive ones. When you have a bad day, don't try to convince yourself it wasn't bad. Instead, recognize that it was bad and congratulate yourself for making it through such a day. That will give you a nice internal reward of serotonin and oxytocin and shut down your losing circuit.

So remember, negative thoughts will happen. That's okay. Just focus on having more positive thoughts.

A NEW VIEW

Many of you will need to change how you view your health journey. Changing anything in life requires focusing on your intentions and motivations, and having a purpose for everything you do. That doesn't mean we won't also be outward focused. We're going to do a deep dive into all things sleep, nutrition, exercise, recovery, and more. But to create sustainable change on the outside, we have to start on the inside. Everything in life begins in your mind—how you view the world around you and the decisions you make. So, from here on, you'll change your outlook in these ways:

- You will not work out, you will *train*. How many times have you gone from one machine to another in a gym, did some random cardio, and then called it a day because you were sweating? After reading this book, you will walk into the gym with one intention—to train toward your goals. You will know what you need to do and how long you need to do it. Gone are the days of going to the gym just to sweat. Every bead of sweat now has a purpose.
- You will not diet, you will *nourish*. Take the negative connotation of dieting out of your mind and instead think about nourishing your body. The true meaning of nutrition is to get nutrients. Everything that goes into your mouth has a purpose: to nourish your body.
- You will not eat, you will *fuel*. How often do you eat when you're not even hungry? We tend to eat when we're bored, stressed, sad, or just because it's technically mealtime. Instead, start thinking about food as fuel. Its purpose is to give us nutrients and energy. Think of it like you do about gas for your car. The amount of gas you need depends on how far you're driving. If you keep putting gas in your tank but never drive far, you'll overfill the tank.
- You will not sleep, you will *replenish*. Sleep is the most important part of your health equation. Your body needs sleep; without it, everything else will fail.

See the difference? Even if you stop reading right now, simple mindset shifts will set you up for success.

MINDSETS, OR THE MINIMUM MENTALITIES

The Minimum Method is about living each day optimally with minimum effort for maximum results. I know some of you will do everything I recommend in the book while others will pick and choose, and that is totally okay. I recognize everyone is different. So I've divided the plan into three different mindsets I call the minimum mentalities. Read the descriptions below and be honest with yourself about which one best describes you. You may be a mix of two or even all three—that's fine! But my hope is that the categories will help you navigate all the advice given throughout the book.

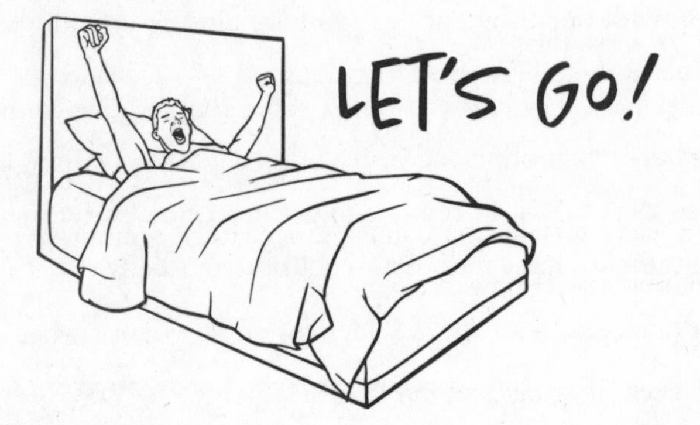

Let's Go! Mindset:

- You get overwhelmed with everything you "should" be doing to optimize your health, causing you to sometimes stop before you even start.
- You want tangible methods that aren't too difficult to understand and are easily integrated into your daily life.
- If we go with the analogy that you must sit up before you can crawl, crawl before you can walk, and walk before you can run, then you're in the sitting up phase.

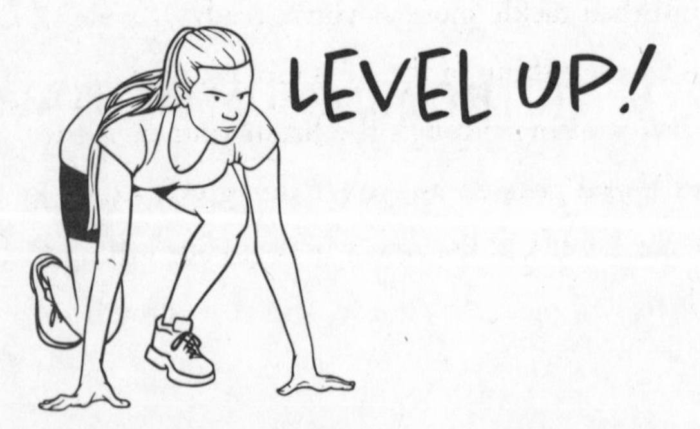

Level Up! Mindset:

- You've tried different diet and exercise plans before—some have worked and others, not so much. Now you're ready for more.
- You don't want to go all out and change every aspect of your life, but you are willing to make some changes to help you reach your goals.
- Keeping with our baby analogy, you are already crawling all over the place and ready to take those first steps.

Max Out! Mindset:

- You are ready to take the major plunge, fully commit to a plan, and stick to it no matter how much change it involves.
- You've been jogging and are ready to start running.

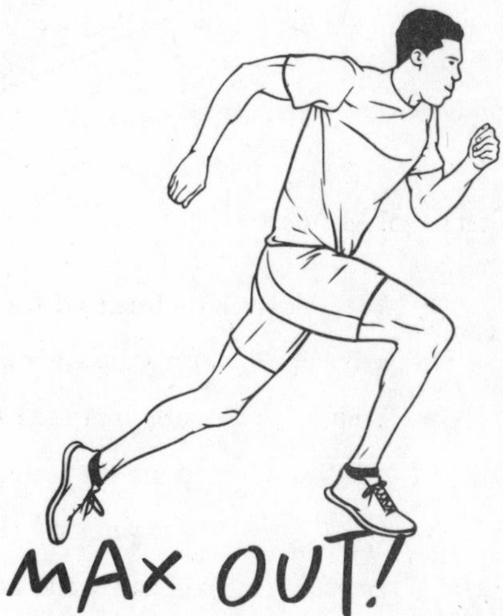

Do you know which one (or two) categories you fit into? Okay, here's how this is going to work. Each chapter will give recommendations for various aspects of life organized by the minimum mentalities. If you fall into the Let's Go! category, you'll start with that list and work through it at your own pace. Start with a couple of changes that feel doable and then tackle more as you're ready. If you're a Level Up! person, then you will do everything in the Let's Go! list plus the recommendations in the Level Up! list, working through the list at your own pace. And if you're ready to Max Out!—you guessed it—you're doing everything in the Let's Go! list, everything in the Level Up! list, and working your way through everything in the Max Out! list.

These categories serve as a guide for how to best utilize the recommendations in this book, but don't feel like you need to stick entirely to one category. Maybe you're more in the Let's Go! camp, but some of the Max Out! sleeping habits seem doable to you. Then go for it! Never hold yourself back because of some label or definition. I want you to see the advice in this book as a healthy buffet, and you have the power to choose how you fill your plate.

2

REST ASSURED, SLEEP MATTERS

SOME PEOPLE SAY, "I'LL SLEEP WHEN I'M DEAD"

You might have assumed the most important chapter would be about food. Nope. Or maybe exercise. Nope. The truth is, my beautiful friends, it's all about sleep. And that's why this chapter is a monster chapter (they won't all be this long!). If you only read and implement the strategies in one chapter of this book, it should be this one. Sleeping is by far the most important when it comes to your overall health and longevity. I highly recommend you read the entire chapter so you have a better understanding of sleep—how it works and why it's so important. But if you don't have time for that, you can flip to the end of the chapter for a down and dirty list of Minimum Method sleep protocols.

In the early days of my career, people would talk about the importance of exercise for good health in one sentence and then the importance of diet in another, never fusing them together. Then finally people started to talk about diet and exercise combined. That's closer to the truth but still not quite right. Here's the truth: sleep, diet, and exercise, in that order, are important to good health. That's right—sleep is the absolute most important, nutrition second, and then exercise. I realize that may come as a shock, considering I make a living telling people to lift weights, but it's true. Let me make my case.

Are you a parent? If so, think back to the early days of parenting and how you felt after days and weeks with little to no sleep. If you're not a parent, ask any new parent how they're feeling. Or think back to how you felt the last time you got very little sleep.

When my son was born, I took two weeks off work to enjoy him and help my wife as much as I could. Let's be honest—moms do most of the work in the beginning, especially if they're breastfeeding. Our son would eat every couple of hours and wake up at all hours of the night. My wife and I were like walking zombies with a case of looming narcolepsy. When I returned to work a couple of weeks later, my sleep-deprived mind wasn't as sharp, my energy was extremely low, and I struggled during my training to lift the lighter weights I used to use to warm up. You see, I had been operating on an extreme lack of sleep and really had no idea how it would affect my mind and my body. No amount of coffee or proper eating could make up for my lack of sleep. Sadly—and too often—that is how we live our everyday lives. We are wired and tired.

The importance of sleep is too often overlooked, and that's an absolute shame. How many times have you heard someone say—or you have said it yourself—that they'll sleep when they're dead? It's a popular saying, and I cringe every time I hear one of my clients say it. Honestly, it's the dumbest thing I've ever heard, especially when talking about trying to get your ideal body.

I SAY, "I WILL DIE FASTER, BE DUMBER, AND HAVE LESS ENERGY IF I DON'T SLEEP"

Sleep is essential to every single facet of our lives. If we don't sleep well—and there is a difference between getting enough sleep and getting good sleep—we pay the price.

As a certified sleep science coach, I've studied this topic in depth. And to be honest, I didn't really believe in the profound effects getting good sleep could have on me until I really focused on my sleep hygiene. So yes, I do in fact practice what I preach. As I write this book, I'm thirty-nine years old—I'll pause for you to comment on how good I look for my age ;-)—and I feel (and look!) the best I've ever felt thanks to finally prioritizing my sleep. And I've never had this much energy. Let's look at why sleep is so critical.

Sleep Affects Your Self-Control

Not getting enough quality sleep is like smoking a joint. And yes, you read that correctly—like smoking a joint. Think of the last time you had a bad night of sleep. I'm willing to bet that the next day you craved foods that are have a high taste reward but low nutritional value (think Cheetos). The day after a poor night of sleep is like having the munchies. You crave foods you would normally have the willpower to avoid, like donuts, ice cream, chips, you get the point. For me it's like being back in college when I wasn't getting enough sleep and maybe also had the legit munchies.

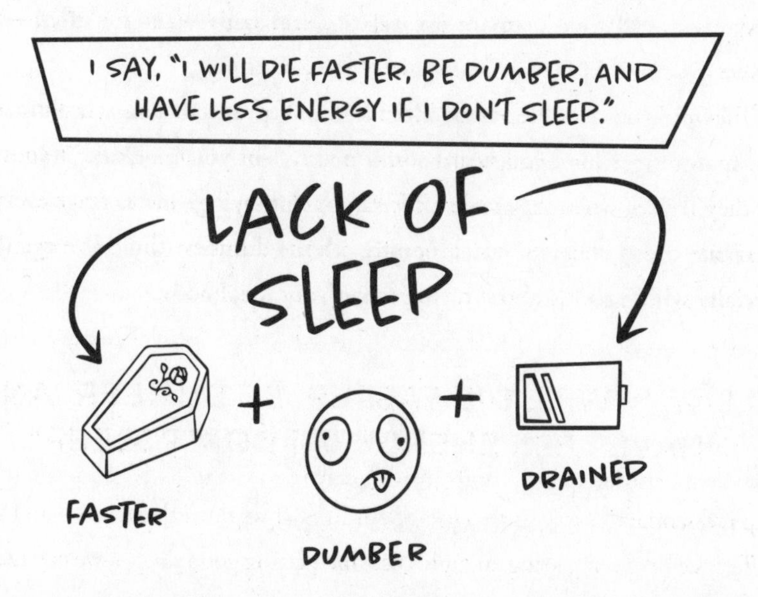

There's even research to back up this bad sleep–munchie theory. A study from the University of Chicago compared food cravings between people who got eight and a half hours of sleep to people who only got four and a half hours of sleep. The group who got less sleep experienced a decreased ability to control their desires when snack foods were placed in front of them.[1]

There's also basic body chemistry involved. Ghrelin is a hormone in your body involved with hunger, whereas leptin is a hormone that helps make you feel full. What impacts these hormone levels? Lots of things do, but a big one is sleep. When you don't get enough sleep, your ghrelin levels rise and your leptin levels go down. Even one night of poor sleep can cause you to crave[2] up to 20 percent more calories[3] the next day. That means you feel hungrier, but what you really need is sleep.

Sleep Affects Your Weight

The less sleep you get, the more fat you carry.[4] That's a bold statement, I know, but several studies have looked at the correlation between the amount of sleep someone gets and the amount of body fat they store, usually surrounding the midsection.[5] Studies even took lifestyle factors, demographics, and work into account and still found an inverse relationship between hours of sleep and pounds of fat.[6] And it gets worse.

If you are on a calorie-controlled diet and trying to lose weight—ideally from fat—not getting enough sleep will make that a lot more difficult.[7] That's because a lack of sleep negatively affects your nutrient partitioning. That means the nutrients you consume won't be properly used by your body for repair and energy but will more likely be stored as fat. Any weight loss you experience will come from precious—and metabolically active—lean muscle tissue that you'd much rather keep.

If I've said it once, I've said it a million times—more muscle equals higher metabolism, more energy, more insulin sensitivity (this is a good thing), and many other benefits that help with the aging process.

Not getting enough sleep triggers the body to store more fat. Remember ghrelin, our hunger hormone? Well, it also promotes fat storage. So less sleep equals higher ghrelin levels and more fat storage. Sleep also affects cortisol and insulin levels, which deal with fat storage. On top of that, not getting enough sleep causes stress, which results in increased fat usually around the midsection (a.k.a. visceral fat surrounding the abdominal organs, omentum fat like an apron of fat tissue under the abdominal muscles, and subcutaneous fat that we can physically grab between the skin and abdominal wall).

Sleep Affects Your Brain

Not sleeping enough will make you dumber. Yes, I said it, and I'm sure you can relate. Have you ever had a bad night's sleep—or worse, a couple of bad nights in a row—and then had to use your brain the next morning? When it comes to cognitive reasoning or problem solving, your brain is mush when it doesn't get enough sleep. Again, there is research to back this up. One study had a group solve problems of varying degrees of difficulty. When that group got less sleep, they struggled with the more difficult problems, while there was no difference solving the easy ones.[8]

Lack of sleep also causes us to forget a lot. When we sleep, our brains consolidate what we learned during the day, our experiences and memories, deciding what needs to be remembered (filed to long-term storage) and what can be thrown out. If we don't get enough sleep, that process can't fully happen, and our short-term memory is seriously affected.

Another important process happens while we sleep—cerebrospinal fluid washes through our brains to clear out any toxins. This is an important point for all the people out there who say they are fine on only six hours of sleep or less. There are always exceptions to rules and strange anomalies, so I'm not saying these people are totally wrong. But an overwhelming body of evidence points to a higher risk of health problems after years and years of getting little sleep.[9] This is likely due to the brain-washing process. The cumulative effect of sleep deprivation is that your brain can't fully clear itself out, and that adds up over the years.

So unless you are getting some sort of award for being a lack-of-sleep warrior, do yourself a favor and get more rest.

It is estimated that 2 to 9 percent of adults in the United States have sleep apnea, with most of them going undiagnosed.[10] Sleep apnea is a serious matter. In addition to disrupting your sleep—and all the negative consequences that come from that—it also doubles your risk of Alzheimer's.[11] Why? Because when we sleep, cerebrospinal fluid washes toxins out of our brain, and that includes the plaque involved with Alzheimer's. That plaque starts to build up twenty to thirty years prior to the onset of Alzheimer's, so your sleep habits today directly affect your risk of Alzheimer's. If you think you could have sleep apnea, participate in a sleep study. And if you already know you have sleep apnea, get a continuous positive airway pressure (CPAP) machine ASAP.

Sleep Affects Your Mood

A lack of sleep can make you feel depressed. This is one effect that I am all too familiar with. If you follow me on social media (@joeythurmanfit, for a shameless plug) or have listened to my TEDx talk, then you know that I've struggled with depression since I was a teenager. When I don't get enough sleep, I notice my depression creeping back, which it's not surprising. A lack of sleep has been shown to produce a neural wave pattern that is often observed with depression.[12] You are likely to feel sadder and have less of a positive outlook on life and your own self-worth when you don't get enough sleep.

Sleep Affects Your Health

This may sound obvious at this point, so I'll get more specific. Not getting enough sleep increases your risk of metabolic syndrome.[13] Metabolic syndrome is a combination of issues that leads to an overall decline of your health.

Metabolic syndrome often includes the following conditions:

- Insulin resistance: The cells in your liver, muscles, and fat don't respond well to glucose/sugar and can't be used for energy. This is likely to lead to prediabetes and type 2 diabetes.
- Hypertension: High blood pressure.
- Obesity: Cis males with a body fat of 26 percent or higher and cis females with a body fat of 34 percent or higher.

In terms of insulin resistance specifically, the importance of sleep is no joke. Sleeping two hours less per night when compared to seven hours over the course of only one week can induce a state of insulin resistance.[14] Furthermore, only one night of four hours or less of sleep induces insulin resistance.[15] That means you crave more sugary foods, and your body is less able to use those sugars so it will store them as fat instead.

All the above effects of sleep deprivation create a cycle. You don't sleep well, which makes you feel fatigued the next day, resulting in you making poor decisions and being hungrier, meaning you probably eat like crap and don't train, plus you feel down, and then all that snowballs into another bad night of sleep.

Poor sleep is so bad for your health that it's finally getting the attention it deserves from the medical community, and not just from doctors who specialize in sleep. A 2019 study published in the *Journal of Internal Medicine* coined the term *circadian syndrome* to describe all the health issues that come from not getting enough sleep.[16] The researchers looked at the effects of disturbances to the circadian system. We'll discuss your circadian system a little later in the chapter, but basically it regulates pretty much every aspect of your metabolism and your health. The researchers feel so strongly about the importance of a healthy circadian system that they've actually proposed changing the name *metabolic syndrome* to *circadian syndrome* and treating it with circadian medicine. This treatment would include light exposure and the timing of working out, eating, taking certain medications, and sleeping.

My point? This is just the beginning of our understanding of how important sleep is for our overall health and happiness.

WHAT EXACTLY IS SLEEP?

Matthew Walker, PhD, is a neuroscientist, psychologist, professor, and basically the greatest sleep expert currently alive. If you ever want to do a deep dive into sleep, start listening to any of the many podcasts he's been interviewed on or read his book, *Why We Sleep: Unlocking the Power of Sleep and Dreams*. One of my favorite quotes of his is "the brain paralyzes the body so the mind can sleep." Think about it—when do our minds ever get to rest? They're "on" all day, non-stop. We tend to think of sleep as a time for the bodies to rest, but even more so, it's a time for our minds to get some much needed rest.

Here's a quick, CliffsNotes-type list of some of the incredible benefits that come from sleep:

- Our immune system strengthens. Proper sleep increases our bodies' T cells' functions, which destroy cells that have been infected by viruses and other pathogens.[17]
- Blood flow increases, bringing oxygen and nutrients to our tissues and muscles, allowing them to recover, repair, and regenerate cells.
- We gain better control over our fears and emotions. The amygdala is the part of the brain responsible for fears. When we are well rested, our amygdala is better able to respond to stressful events in a more controlled way. When we don't get enough sleep, our emotions and fears can get the best of us. Sleep can quite literally help your mental health.[18]

All of these benefits happen at different stages throughout sleep. That's why getting enough sleep and enough quality sleep is important—you need to get through all the stages to reap the benefits.

Sleep ultimately can be broken down into two main categories: REM (rapid eye movement) and non-REM. During non-REM sleep, we save our memories, regulate our heart rates and blood pressures, and restore our autonomic nervous system. REM sleep, on the other hand, is like therapy. It helps us better regulate our emotions, and our dreams help us work through things we have on our minds. Studies have also shown that not getting enough REM sleep increases the risk for all causes of mortality.

If you want to get even more detailed, there are technically five different stages of sleep. Stages 1 through 4 are non-REM sleep and stage 5 is REM sleep. Furthermore, stages 1 and 2 are considered light non-REM, and stages 3 and 4 are deep non-REM.

Stages 1 and 2: Light Sleep

The first stage is so light that if you wake up, you may not think you were asleep, and waking up during this stage is the least disruptive to your night's sleep. Light sleep is just as important as all the other stages of sleep. Both your heart rate and breathing slow down. Electrical activity in your brain helps its communication system better learn and remember information. About half of your night's sleep is spent in the light stage of sleep. In the second stage, your heart rate slows even more, and your body temperature starts to drop. This is preparing you for deep sleep.

Stages 3 and 4: Deep Sleep

In stages three and four, you begin to enter what is known as slow-wave sleep. Your body becomes motionless, your breathing rate decreases, and your blood pressure drops. This is when tissue healing occurs, your immune system strengthens, and your muscles receive an increased supply of blood and growth hormones.

Stage 5: REM Sleep

The final and deepest stage of sleep is the REM stage. You typically enter this stage of sleep around ninety minutes after you fall asleep. And that's when your brain paralyzes your body so you are allowed to dream without your body acting out. While REM sleep tends to get credit for dreams, you can actually dream in all stages of sleep. Your dreams are just longer and more story-like in REM sleep.

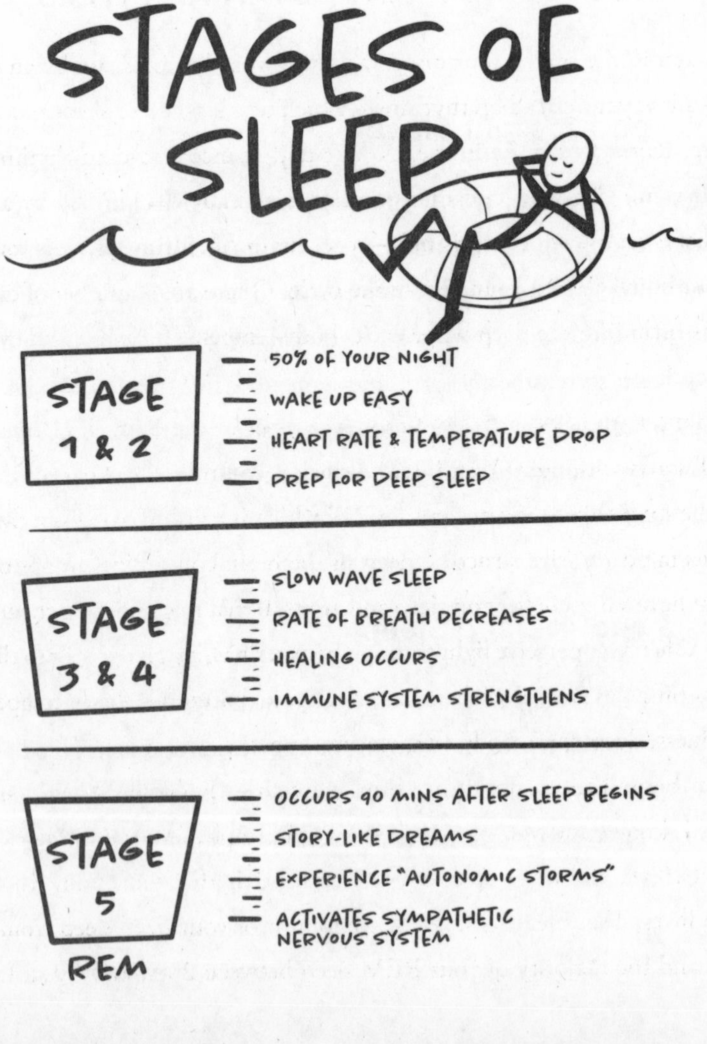

During REM sleep, your body goes through autonomic storms, where your heart rate drops and then drastically rises to activate the sympathetic nervous system. These storms can have some fun results for the sleeper (think wet dreams for both cis men and cis women).

A full sleep cycle—going through all five stages—typically takes between 90 and 110 minutes. A clue that you've gone through a full sleep cycle is when you roll over or readjust yourself in bed. It's a sign you've finished your REM sleep so your body is no longer paralyzed and now wants to move and reposition before another cycle begins. Ideally, we go through four to six cycles per night.

WHETHER YOU CAN DANCE OR NOT, YOU'VE GOT CIRCADIAN RHYTHMS

Sleep starts in the brain. Your body, including your brain, is run by an internal clock—a.k.a. your circadian rhythms—which tells it when to sleep and when to wake up. (*Circadian* in Latin means "one day," hence circadian rhythm is one day's rhythm.) But your circadian rhythm is actually determined by a master clock that is set by—not surprisingly—your brain. So, ultimately, it is your brain (not your body) setting your sleep-wake cycle. (There are a number of circadian rhythms including the sleep-wake cycle, body-temperature cycle, and even hormonal cycle.)

What sets the clock? As with most processes in the body, it's complicated, but it all starts with light. Your internal clock is controlled by a part of the brain called the suprachiasmatic nucleus (SCN), which is a group of cells in the hypothalamus (a peanut-size structure deep in the brain containing groups of nerve cells that have a direct effect on sleep and arousal) that responds to light and dark signals. When you perceive light through your retinas, a signal is sent to the SCN that sets off a cascade of events that affect your hormones, body temperature, wakefulness, sleep drive, body temperature, appetite, and more.

Your body likes to stay in rhythm as much as possible. When you go off rhythm, it knows and you pay the price. For example, let's say you typically go to bed at 10 PM and wake up at 6 AM. That's the rhythm your body knows and (maybe) loves. That means you are getting most of your deep sleep from 10 PM to 2 AM and the majority of your REM sleep between 2 AM and 6 AM. Let's say you have a big party night or have to work or study super late one night and for whatever reason, you stay up until 2 AM. Logically, you'd think that you would just be starting your entire sleep cycle later and that you'd go through the normal stages, just starting at 2 AM instead of 10 PM. Nope. Somehow your body knows that 2 AM is when you typically get your REM sleep so it will spend less time in the first couple of sleep stages—and pretty much all your deep sleep—and just go right into REM sleep. REM sleep is great and important, but so is all that restorative deep sleep that you miss out on that night.

Here's an example of an average circadian cycle for someone who goes to bed around 11 PM and wakes around 7 AM:

- 3 AM to 7 AM: Your energy will be at its lowest.
- 4:30 AM: Body temperature is at its lowest point to make sure REM sleep occurs.
- 6:45 AM: Blood pressure spikes to prepare you to wake up.
- 7:30 AM: Melatonin secretion stops.
- 8:30 AM: Your bowels get moving.
- 9 AM: Testosterone is at its highest to wake you up.
- 10 AM to 1 PM: High amounts of energy and alertness.
- 1 to 3 PM: Might get an afternoon slump.
- 2:30 PM: Coordination at its highest.
- 3:30 PM: Faster reaction times.
- 5 PM: Best cardio efficiency and muscular strength.
- 9 PM: Melatonin starts to rise to wind you down.
- 10:30 PM: Bowel movements are slowed down so you don't poop yourself at night.

If you are a shift worker, you are at a higher risk of developing circadian misalignment. Follow these steps to minimize the risk:

- Try to make sure your night mimics a normal day.
- Get light when you first wake up either via the sun or artificial light.

- Avoid coffee at least six hours before going to bed.
- Get your workout in earlier in the day to set your clock.
- Your bedroom should mimic nighttime even if it's daylight out. Make sure it is as dark as possible and around 65 degrees Fahrenheit.

Sleep procrastination, or revenge bedtime, refers to purposely pushing back your bedtime to give yourself more time for activities such as relaxing, watching TV, or hanging out with your significant other. People who have busy lives and are juggling stressful jobs, children, and other responsibilities will often delay going to bed to give themselves more "me time." On the surface, this makes total sense and seems like a good idea. The problem is that those people usually can't also push back their wake up time. So ultimately they are decreasing their overall sleep time. And, as I hope you understand by now, not getting enough sleep is never a good idea.

Here's a Minimum Method tip. Say you like watching a movie or a show before bed. Record that show, and instead of staying up late, watch it at some other point, even if it's ten minutes at a time on your phone while going to the bathroom (I know we all do this!). The goal is to make sure that your "me time" doesn't leave you tired.

Now, if that show is scary or full of action, I especially don't want you watching it before bed as this will likely cause your system to go into a sympathetic state and make it harder to fall asleep.

Understanding your circadian rhythm is important for all areas of your life and health. You want to make sure you're timing certain activities to work with your circadian rhythm, not against it. For example, working out too close to your bedtime can increase your adrenaline and make it harder for you to fall asleep. Taking certain medications and supplements can affect how fast you can fall asleep and even how well you stay asleep. Eating too close to your bedtime can make it harder to fall asleep because your body is still working to digest your food so it can't shift into relaxation mode. That's one of the reasons that in chapter five, I'm going to tell you to eat carbs at night.

IT'S NOT ALL CIRCADIAN RHYTHM; OTHER BIOLOGICAL FACTORS ARE INVOLVED TOO

Outside of your circadian rhythm, there are biological factors at play that impact when you sleep and when you wake. Our biology is almost eerily tied to the planet. So much of our sleep and wake cycle is intertwined with the rising and setting of the sun.

Let's pretend you don't need to use an alarm clock to wake up (and maybe some of you don't). Usually within one to three hours of the sun rising, your body naturally generates an internal signal to trigger certain hormones to make you wake up, namely cortisol, adrenaline, and epinephrine. Pretty cool, huh? So the best way to maximize your sleep and your awake time is to align your circadian rhythm with the sun as much as possible. But let's be honest—that isn't always easy.

For example, most people don't have the luxury of being able to wake up naturally. They have to rely on an alarm clock, which is like a shortcut that ultimately triggers a lot of the same responses, such as a spike in cortisol, as the rising sun. The problem is that the sudden burst of noise results in much more cortisol than is needed to wake up. Don't worry. That doesn't mean you're screwed because you have to use an alarm clock. You have two options to prevent or undo the negative effects of an alarm clock:

1. Use an alarm clock with an alarm that gradually increases in noise (or light).
2. Take a minute after your alarm goes off to calm yourself down. Sit on the side of your bed and take some deep breaths, maybe recite a mantra—whatever will help.

If your alarm goes off before the sun is up and you're waking up in a dark room, there isn't enough light to trigger some important reactions. Again, that doesn't mean you're out of luck. Here are some other ways you can let your body know it's time to wake up:

- Walk around
- Drink some water

- Exercise
- Take a sip of apple cider vinegar

Okay, so now that you're up and your day has started, what makes you get sleepy? A little thing called adenosine. Adenosine is a chemical in your body—actually present in all your cells—that builds up throughout the day and creates sleep hunger. It is completely independent of your internal clock. In the morning, your adenosine levels are very low and the longer you are awake, the more it builds up. Adenosine peaks around twelve to sixteen hours after you wake up.

Now let's talk about melatonin. When people think of melatonin, they generally think of something exogenous, like a pill. But melatonin is naturally occurring in our bodies and an important part of our circadian rhythm cycle. In humans, melatonin is secreted from our enigmatic pineal gland during the night. This gland is responsible for sensing light-dark cycles in our environment. When it senses darkness, it produces and secretes melatonin to help us sleep. This is why it's so important to be aware of how much light you get and when you get it. Remember, we are tied to the planet and the sun. Your eyes are sensitive to light from above because it's similar to the sun. Too much light at night will interfere with your melatonin.[19]

Generally, higher levels of melatonin are released two hours before bedtime, with peak levels around 3 to 4 AM, and then they start to wane. That's why you wake up a little sleepier if you get up earlier than normal—your melatonin is still waning. And waning melatonin can affect more than just your alertness—it can affect your food choices and insulin sensitivity (more on this in chapter five).

EVERYONE HAS A DIFFERENT INTERNAL CLOCK

Would you consider yourself a morning person? A night owl? Something in between? This is where sleep gets really interesting—those personas legitimately exist. We are all wired a little bit differently when it comes to when we like to sleep. Some people truly are morning people and will never stay up past 10 PM, whereas others can't wake up before 10 AM. There is no right or wrong—they're just different.

Sleep experts have identified four different sleep chronotypes, or internal clocks: bear, wolf, lion, and dolphin. People of each chronotype go to sleep, wake up, and even are productive at different times of the day. If you want to dive deeper into sleep chronotypes, there is no shortage of information on the internet. But here's a quick rundown.

Sadly, most of society is built around the 9 AM–5 PM work schedule, which works fine if you're a bear. But for the late-sleeping wolves, nap-needing lions, and sleep-lacking dolphins, it can be a struggle to focus and be productive during the defined work day. Knowing your chronotype can help you determine when you should do certain activities and how to optimize your productivity. For example, if you're a wolf, stop trying to wake up early to work out. You're just setting yourself up for failure. Instead, you're fine to exercise after work because you'll have plenty of time to unwind before you go to sleep.

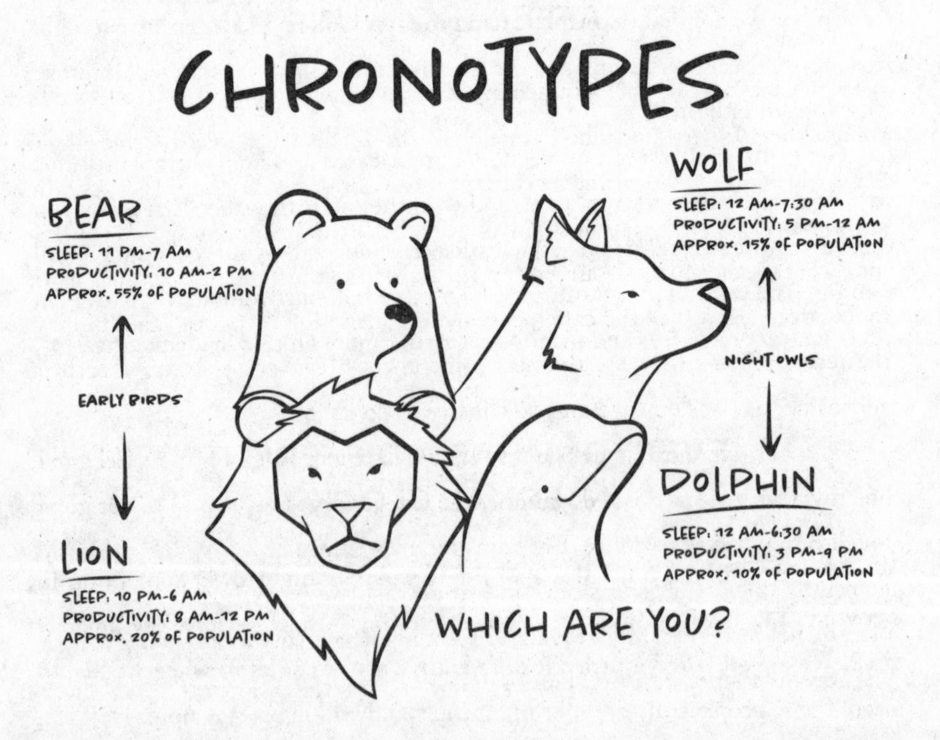

No matter what your current circadian rhythm or sleep chronotype, here's the good news—you're not locked into it. Our bodies are resilient and our internal clock can be changed with some effort. You are not stuck with your chronotype. It will take some time—and there will be an adjustment period—but you can train your body to be on the sleep schedule that makes the most sense for your life.

While there are many mechanisms involved in setting your internal clock, when you want to reset it, light is going to be your best friend. Working with natural light will be the easiest and quickest way to take control of your circadian rhythm.

If you want to start waking up earlier, you need light exposure earlier, before you wake up. That means open up those curtains and get that light in your room as early as possible. Or if you're trying to wake up before the sun rises, you can use artificial light. Consider getting a sunrise alarm clock, which will slowly light up your room, simulating a sunrise.

THE CAFFEINE CONUNDRUM

All right, I know there are a bunch of coffee lovers reading this book so let's talk about caffeine. First, here's how caffeine works—it acts like an adenosine antagonist, blocking the adenosine receptor so it can't build up. Caffeine isn't actually a stimulant in and of itself; it simply blocks the sleepy signal that makes you feel more awake and allows your body's natural stimulants (like dopamine) work more effectively. Once the caffeine wears off, adenosine can once again bind to the receptor. This is where the post-caffeine crash can come from—a rush of adenosine that was blocked and now is free to do its job.

Caffeine does have some benefits. It gives us energy and makes us feel good, literally. Caffeine increases dopamine, the feel-good chemical. So I'm not going to tell you to quit your coffee. But I am going to tell you how to make sure it isn't negatively impacting your sleep. And to do that, we have to look at the entire picture, not just your ability to fall asleep at night, but your ability to wake up as well. Seems counterintuitive, but it's not.

If you are a coffee drinker, I want you to wait sixty to ninety minutes after you've woken up to have a cup of coffee. Drinking coffee any sooner may interfere with your body's natural cortisol levels and cause you to need more caffeine sooner. Waiting lets your body activate its natural wake-up processes and lets the coffee give you sustained energy throughout the day.

The next rule is no caffeine after noon. Why? Because caffeine has a half-life of six to eight hours. You don't want any caffeine left in your system when your body starts to relax in preparation for going to sleep. If you have caffeine lingering in your system, your sleep will be light instead of deep, and it will mess up your non-REM to REM ratio that night.

Another not-so-fun fact about caffeine is that it tends to affect cis women more than men. Sorry ladies. But you don't have certain enzymes that aid in breaking down caffeine so you metabolize it more slowly than your cis male counterparts.

Again, I'm not going to tell you to put away your coffee cup forever. But I would be remiss not to share one more little tidbit about coffee. Did you know you can build up a tolerance to coffee when you drink it regularly? That's because over time your brain actually changes and creates more adenosine receptors to try to compete with all the caffeine. So even more caffeine is needed to block all the receptors so you feel awake. An unfortunate side effect is that your brain also decreases the number of norepinephrine (a natural stimulant) receptors, making you even more dependent on caffeine to feel energized. So my take on coffee is that—as with most things—moderation is key.

LET'S TALK ALCOHOL

Alcohol is extremely misunderstood when it comes to its relationship with sleep. Many people turn to alcohol to help them fall asleep. And how many of you have used the phrase *passed out* when talking about sleeping after drinking just a little too much (my hand is raised right now)? Here's the thing with alcohol. Yes, it will help you fall asleep, but there's a trade-off. Your sleep will be less restful, and you'll have less REM sleep.

That being said, alcohol can have some benefits when it comes to your sleep. If you have a stressful day and a glass of wine or something will help you relax into your parasympathetic nervous system (a.k.a. de-stress), then go for it. Just don't have too much because then it will mess with your sleep.

Okay, but what happens when you go to a party or have a night out and you have a little too much and all you want to do is sleep the next day? As tempting as it is, try not to. The better decision is to get up and go about your normal routine, then go to sleep at your normal time.

THE TRUTH ABOUT SLEEP AIDS & SUPPLEMENTS

Time to talk about another popular sleep subject—sleep aids and supplements. Sleep aids like Ambien, Lunesta, or Sonata work to boost production of a neurotransmitter known as gamma-aminobutyric acid (GABA). GABA helps to quiet down or make certain nerve cells called neurons in our brains sleepy. The problem with sleep aids is that they make you drowsy but don't allow you to get proper REM sleep because they restrict the deep brain waves during REM.

It's similar to passing out drunk. Just because you are knocked on your ass unconscious does not mean you got good sleep! Lots of people who take these sleep aids often wake up groggy and then get in a car to drive to work, which is not a good combination. Taking these sleep aids can lead to over-caffeinating yourself the morning after, not utilizing your cortisol wake cycle, and then getting that adenosine flood when the coffee wears off, making you even more tired in the afternoon.

Essentially, sleep aids mess with your natural sleep balance and processes and ultimately make you dependent on them for sleep. I recommend tapering off them if possible and trying some of the more natural solutions we'll discuss at the end of this chapter.

One final waning about sleep aids—these drugs (Ambien, Lunesta, and Sonata) have received a black box warning by the FDA due to multiple cases of semiconscious behavior such as sleepwalking or driving while sleeping that resulted in serious injury or death.

On the other hand, some supplements are much less harmful and can be helpful for some people:

- Melatonin can help you fall asleep, but know that it won't help you stay asleep. Be cautious when taking melatonin. Studies have shown that the amount of melatonin listed on a label is not always accurate, and there could be more or less actual melatonin present in the supplement.[20]
- Magnesium is a natural way to increase neurotransmitters like GABA that help the mind relax and drift off to sleep. A lot of people are deficient in magnesium, but before you start supplementing, you should see if you're getting enough from your food. The recommended dietary allowance for magnesium is 360–420 milligrams per day. Foods with high levels of magnesium include pumpkin seeds, flax seeds, almonds, and spinach.

  You should track your magnesium intake from your food for about a week before deciding to supplement. If you need to take magnesium supplements, be careful as they can cause some GI distress. Start with around 200 milligrams per day and see how your stomach handles it before increasing the dosage. You may even consider taking Epsom salt baths, as some studies suggest you can absorb magnesium through the skin.[21]
- Theanine can help take away jitters from energy drinks consumed too close to bedtime. Theanine has been shown to have a calming effect and can even help with anxiety.[22] There is no standard dose, but most research recommends around 200–400 milligrams a day.
- Apigenin is a natural herb that can help your muscles relax. The antioxidant is found in chamomile tea and is what helps give the tea its calming effect.[23]
- CBD and THC in small doses can help you calm down, but know that too much will negatively affect your sleep cycle.

- Valerian root is a plant that can help you fall asleep and has been shown to help overall mood the following day. Look for supplements that have 450 milligrams of valerian extract standardized for 0.8 to 1 percent valerenic acids.[24]
- Kava root is a plant that can help you relax and calm down (similar to Valium) and can promote sleep quality without a disruption in REM.[25] Extended use of kava may make it less effective, though, so use it sparingly.

Nature has already produced several plants and roots to help you sleep. I always recommend people try something natural first. If you clean up your sleep routine, try these natural herbs and supplements, and if you still have trouble sleeping, it's probably time to see a sleep doctor.

TO NAP OR NOT TO NAP, THAT IS THE QUESTION

When we talk about napping, it's important to remember three points we've discussed so far:

1. Everyone's circadian rhythm is different.
2. There are different sleep chronotypes.
3. Adenosine builds up while we are awake and decreases while we sleep.

Keeping all that in mind, napping is not inherently bad. In fact, one could easily argue that we were designed to nap. My stance on napping is that as long as it doesn't interfere with your ability to fall asleep at your bedtime, so you get enough sleep during the night, then go for it. For most people, that means napping earlier in the day so adenosine has time to build back up. Napping in the afternoon usually means you won't be able to fall asleep at your normal time.

You also want to monitor how long you nap. Remember, a typical sleep cycle is ninety minutes, so ninety minutes is a good length for a nap. If you go longer than that, you start another cycle and unless you can nap for three hours, you'll end up waking up mid-cycle. Plus, the longer the nap, the more your adenosine levels drop.

The main takeaway is to pay attention to how you feel after a nap and how it affects the rest of your day. If you feel good and you're able to still fall asleep at night on time, then nap every day for all I care. But if you feel groggy the rest of the day or can't fall asleep that night, then whatever time you napped that day—or however long your nap was—doesn't work for you.

You also don't have to actually nap to get some of the benefits of napping. There is a concept called non-sleep deep rest that can be very restorative. It's basically resting with your eyes closed without falling asleep. This could be meditating or it could be as simple as just lying in a quiet place removed from external stimulation. As with all health advice, find what works for your body and your schedule.

THE NEVER-ENDING DEBATE: HOW MUCH SLEEP DO YOU REALLY NEED?

The best sleep goal is to program yourself to wake up with the rising sun and go to sleep soon after the sun sets. But that's just not possible for everyone, especially during certain times of the year. So another good rule of thumb is to try to go to sleep at around 10 PM and wake up at around 6 AM. But if you can get to bed earlier, do it! It's hypothesized that every hour of sleep prior to 10 PM is equivalent to two hours of sleep after midnight when the deeper stages occur.

On average, adults need seven to eight hours of sleep per night. But that truly is an average. How much sleep you need is impacted by genetics, age, and your sleep chronotype. And your sleep needs can change over time. Babies require a lot more sleep than adults, and older adults often need less sleep than younger adults. So rather than tell you a set number of hours of sleep to get each night, I'm going to tell you to pay attention to your body and find your individual sleep need.

The easiest way to tell that you're getting enough sleep is when you wake up without an alarm clock. When you require an alarm to wake you up, you are most likely waking up before your body is naturally ready to, and therefore starting the day with a sleep deficit. I realize that might be frustrating news for some of you, and you're thinking there's no way you'll ever be able to wake up naturally to get to the gym, get to work, get the kids to school, and so on.

If your wake-up time isn't negotiable, then try experimenting with your bedtime. And remember, there are a couple factors that play into your total number of hours of sleep: your sleep cycle (Are you waking up before a cycle is finished?) and your circadian rhythm (Does your body know when it's time to sleep and wake?).

Keep in mind that going to bed earlier isn't always the answer. You may need to push your bedtime up a bit. Not the advice you were expecting, I know! But here's an example. Let's say your sleep cycle is ninety minutes. That means that sleeping seven-and-a-half hours will give you five full cycles—that's great! But if you're going to bed eight hours before you have to wake up, you'll have already started another cycle when your alarm goes off. Unless you can go to bed early enough to fit in another full cycle (meaning nine hours of sleep), you're better off going to bed thirty minutes later to get seven and a half hours of sleep and avoid waking up mid-cycle.

> For an exercise to help you find your ideal amount of sleep, go to joeythurman.com/homework.

Finding your sleep cycle isn't the full answer. You also need to pay attention to how you feel throughout the day and over time. Keeping with the example above, where your sleep cycle is hypothetically ninety minutes, you may feel okay getting only six hours of sleep. After all, six hours of sleep doesn't have you waking up mid-cycle. But then how do you feel as the day goes on? Do you get really tired in the late afternoon? Over time, does your brain feel foggy and do you have trouble remembering things? These are all signs that six hours of sleep isn't really enough for you.

If you home in on a bedtime that ensures you are getting enough total sleep and not waking up mid–sleep cycle, and you stick to that bedtime and wake-up time, eventually you should start to naturally wake up before your alarm.

In general, we go through several cycles of sleep per night, and each REM stage gets longer throughout the night until the morning approaches. Those cycles should leave you feeling refreshed and ready to go when you wake up. If they don't, it's time to look at what you're doing throughout the day.

HOW TO WAKE UP

We've talked about falling asleep and waking up with an alarm. Now it's time to discuss waking up naturally. Remember, it's all about creating a healthy circadian rhythm, and that involves not only how you go to sleep, but also how you wake up and even everything in between, which we'll get to next.

Light exposure first thing in the morning is critical. Light suppresses melatonin and triggers all your body's wake-up processes. Light in the morning is best because once the sun is overhead, the quality of light changes. If you can, walk outside in the morning and look toward the sun. If you can't walk outside, looking out the window will suffice.

If you wake up before the sun, artificial light can do the trick. Our neurons don't know the difference between artificial light and sunlight. They only know the difference between low light and bright light. Blue light and yellow light are your best bets to help you wake up, but before you even think it—no, don't use your phone for your blue light source after you first wake up. Your phone is full of emails, texts, news updates, social media alerts, and a slew of other stress-inducing notifications. Your mindset is at its most vulnerable point first thing in the morning. The negative effects of what's in your phone far outweigh the benefits of blue light exposure. It also won't give you enough blue light. Instead, you can use a selfie ring light.

Blue light has been getting a bad rep lately, but it's not always bad. Blue light is actually the closest light to UV on the light spectrum. That's why you want to avoid it later in the day when your body needs to be winding down for sleep. But blue light early in the day isn't harmful. So by all means wear your blue light–blocking glasses in the evening, but no need to sport them all day.

Getting light from the sun first thing in the morning triggers your body's natural cortisol pulse. Triggering a cortisol pulse early in the day allows you to be more awake, regulates your body's circadian rhythm, helps control your blood pressure, and even alleviates some mental health disorders, to name a few of the benefits.[26]

If you're able to go outside and it's bright, you only need about thirty to sixty seconds to trigger your body's natural wake-up process. If it's cloudy outside or a miserable winter day, you might need longer, like up to ten minutes. That would be a perfect time to take a short walk. If you can't get early light or you are up before the sun, you can get one of those selfie ring lights (at least 1,000 lux or more) and use that in the morning for the same effect, but it may take up to thirty minutes to trigger a cortisol pulse.[27]

After getting some light exposure, take a few minutes to do some deep breathing or stretching. Then you can look at your phone and get ready for the day.

YOUR DAY SETS UP YOUR NIGHT

Our sleep is highly dependent on how we spend our days. What we do when we are awake will determine if we fall asleep, when we fall asleep, and if we stay asleep.

Get ready for a surprising statement—I want you to stop wearing your sunglasses so much. I know, I know, you think you're going to harm your eyes if you don't. Here's the thing. If you have to squint (either because it's so bright or the sun is bouncing off a reflective surface into your eyes), then yes, wear sunglasses to protect your eyes. But you don't need to wear shades simply because the sun is out. If you're not squinting, you don't need them.

It's important for your circadian rhythm that your eyes be exposed to light throughout the day. Why? Because your body is super smart. As the sun moves throughout the day, you see the light change angles, signaling the time of day to your body and regulating your hormones and other processes involved in determining when you sleep and when you're awake.

As the sun starts to set, you should start slowing down as well. Try looking toward the horizon for a few minutes to help cue your body that bedtime is coming. Also, turn down the overhead lights in your house or use a light dimmer. Overhead light signals a wakeful state instead of one of rest. You could even consider using candles at night (just be careful), which will also save you money on your electricity bill.

So, to wrap up, sleep is an extremely important yet also complicated process that our bodies and brain go through. And both the quality and quantity of our sleep can be impacted by almost everything we do throughout the day.

THE MINIMUM METHOD SLEEP PROTOCOLS

Let's Go!

- Take a short walk outside as the sun is going down and gaze at the horizon. If you can't walk, you can look at the horizon from your home through a window. This will help trigger a relaxed state before you go to bed.
- Don't eat too late. Remember, eating is for fueling, and you don't need to fuel yourself for sleep. Your body needs time to wind down and get ready for sleep, and it can't do that if you're busy digesting food. Remember, every cell in your body has a circadian rhythm. Research from Dr. Satchin Panda, who wrote the book *The Circadian Code* and coined the phrase *time-restricted eating*, shows that your digestive system needs to "sleep." The average meal takes about five hours to pass

through the stomach and reach the small intestine for nutrient absorption. Time-restricted eating means you stop eating a few hours before bed so your organs and GI tract can rest, which will help you sleep better. To allow for proper digestion and cell recovery, try to go twelve to sixteen hours from your last bite of food at night to your first bite of food the following day. I recommend saving your carbs for dinner because they are easier to digest and the glucose crash works to your advantage when going to sleep.

- Start going to bed at a consistent time (within an hour) every single night and waking up at a consistent time (within an hour) to regulate your circadian rhythm.
- Manage your light exposure. Remember, light plays a major role in our biology and when our bodies think we should be awake or asleep. If our brain detects light it thinks is the sun, it will hinder melatonin and delay the onset of sleep. You want to get as little light as possible after 8 PM. Dim your overhead lights (the overhead part makes your body think it is the sun) and try not to look at any screens an hour before bedtime. That means no more checking your phone right before bed! The blue light from the screen is too similar to the sun. If you must look at a screen close to bedtime, do one of the following:
  - Put on blue-light-blocking glasses a couple of hours before bedtime
  - Put your phone in night mode
  - Use an app that blocks out blue light
  - Use candles when it's safe to do so
- Have a bedtime ritual to further help your body prepare for sleep. Maybe it's reading, knitting, or listening to relaxing music—sticking to a pre-bedtime routine will help your body and mind relax and get ready for rest.
- Get into a parasympathetic state. Your bedtime ritual should not include reading work emails, watching scary or action-packed movies, or doing

anything else that will activate your sympathetic nervous system (a.k.a. stress you out). The goal is to move into your parasympathetic nervous system where you can relax. If that requires a glass of wine to wash away your stressful day, then have at it! And if you are still feeling a little amped, deep-breathing exercises are a great way to calm your body down. I'll give some specific breathing exercises in chapter four.

- Lower your body temperature. When you go to sleep, you don't want your core body temperature too high. A low body temperature is important for falling asleep and getting into the deeper sleep stages. That means you should avoid any activities that will raise your core body temperature before bed. Except sex. Sex is okay—you're welcome! But that does mean avoiding workouts. Try to work out in the morning or at least earlier in the evening so your body has time to naturally cool down before you go to bed.
- Create a relaxing sleep environment. Here are the main components to creating a relaxing sleeping environment:
  - Light: The darker, the better. Remove as much light from your bedroom as possible. If you wake up in the middle of the night to use the restroom or for any other reason, don't turn on any lights or check your phone. You don't want any bright light exposure between 11 PM and 4 AM. Even just checking your phone to see the time will wake up your brain.
  - Temperature: The ideal room temperature for sleeping is 65 degrees Fahrenheit, give or take a few degrees.[28] Our body temperature needs to be able to drop while we sleep, and a warm room will prohibit that. Fun fact: Sleeping in a cold room can also help you burn more fat by increasing the levels of the metabolically active brown fat and an increase in the ability to metabolize fat.[29]
  - Noise. The quieter, the better. If you can hear city or neighbor noises in your bedroom, get a noise machine to help drown them

out. For some reason, white noise seems to be the most popular in the noise machine game, but pink noise is actually better. Pink noise has a deeper bass than white noise does, which people often find more soothing than the higher-pitched white noise.[30] You can also turn on nature sounds, as there have been many studies showing that nature sounds help get your body into a parasympathetic state.

— Electronics. The electric and magnetic fields from your electronics can interfere with your melatonin levels.[31] That means keep your phone in another room, and I even recommend turning off your Wi-Fi each night. If you use your phone as an alarm clock, put it on airplane mode.

- If you use an alarm to wake up, simply shut it off and don't look at your phone. If your alarm is your phone, then turn off the alarm and do not unlock your phone.
- First thing in the morning, get outside to take a walk for five to ten minutes. If you don't have time for that, open one of your windows and get some natural light on your face and gaze toward the sun for a few minutes without hurting your eyes. If you're driving to work as the sun comes up, roll your windows down to get your lux rays.
- If you are a morning coffee or caffeine drinker, wait at least an hour before drinking it to give your elevated cortisol a chance to wake you up naturally.

Level Up!

- Avoid spicy foods at dinner. They can increase your body temperature, and you want a low body temperature for sleeping.
- Take a hot shower. This is another body temperature trick. Taking a hot shower before bed will help trigger your body to cool itself down. A nice

relaxing bath will do the trick as well. Add candles for low-level light and lavender or Epsom salt, and you've got your own sleep spa!

- Drink water. Your brain is primarily water so fuel it up before you go seven to eight hours without any water.
- Do some light yoga or stretches before bed to help your body further relax.
- Do some breathing exercises before bed. Don't worry, they don't have to be anything elaborate. You simply focus on your breath. A good one is the 4-7-8 technique developed by Dr. Andrew Weil. Inhale through your nose for a count of four, hold for a count of seven, and exhale through your mouth for a count of eight. Do this for several rounds.
- Use a sleep tracker. Sleep trackers that measure your heart rate can help you determine whether you're getting enough deep sleep.
- Figure out if you are a bear, wolf, lion, or dolphin. Optimize your day (meetings, work, exercise, and so on) around when you will be most productive.

Max Out!

- Watch your omega-6 intake. Too much omega-6 can create inflammation and cause sleep issues.
- Manage allergies. Pollen and other allergens can stick to your clothes and in your hair. If you suffer from allergies, don't change out of your clothes in your room, and be sure to take a shower before bed. Otherwise, the allergens will go to bed with you and make it harder for you to fall and stay asleep.
- Meditate. Meditation helps bring your mind into a parasympathetic state by activating cells and circuits in the body to calm down. A simple body scan or breathing meditation can work wonders to help you sleep. I use an app called BrainTap that has relaxing sounds and talks me

through some guided body scanning and meditation tactics. It usually gets me to fall asleep before the twenty-minute track is up. I download the tracks and turn my phone on airplane mode so my phone doesn't disrupt my sleep.

- Listen to binaural beats. Binaural beats are when you listen to two tones at different frequencies, one in each ear, at the same time. They've been proven to help people relax, especially when using low-frequency beats in the delta, theta, and alpha ranges.

3

BRAIN POWER

Upgrading the Smartest Computer You'll Ever Own

THE BRAIN EXPLAINED: WHY UNDERSTANDING YOUR BRAIN MATTERS

Our brains are much more than squishy think tanks inside our heads. We are walking around with extremely sophisticated "computers" in our heads that have a multitude of functions and are at the root of our intelligence. So again, I recommend you read the whole chapter so you can soak up all this great knowledge about your brain. But if you're short on time (or attention span!), there's a nice to-the-point list of Minimum Method brain protocols at the end of the chapter. Let's dive into the brain.

Your brain receives every sensation your body encounters, processes it, and then communicates its analysis back to your body. For example, you see a car coming toward you. Your brain analyzes what you're seeing, recognizes it as danger, and then tells your legs to walk (or jump!) out of the way. This happens so fast that you take it for granted. Even what is considered natural instinct is still work and processing for your brain.

Every single touch, breath, and emotion that you have has to be processed by your brain. It is by far the most important organ in your entire body. It is also the head of your nervous system, which includes the spinal cord and all the nerves throughout your entire body. By way of the nervous system, your brain controls every aspect of your body.

So basically, your brain is deciding how you see the world, from what you actually see, touch, and feel to how you make sense of it and what you decide to do about it. It truly is creating the world you live in. If you really think about it, you live inside your head. Your life is the narrative that your brain is creating—that's how powerful it is. But it doesn't do this in a vacuum. There are many factors that influence how your mind analyzes and makes sense of the world around you and all the people in it. That's what we're going to dive into in this chapter.

THE BRAIN IN ACTION

Your thoughts can bring you back to the past or project you into the future. But where the rubber really hits the road is with your actions, or behaviors. Actions come in two different forms: intentional and reflexive (or reactionary). An intentional action is when you think about something and then deliberately decide to do it. A reflexive action is when you do something without thinking about it, such as when you blink, breathe, or scratch an itch.

Here's the thing. Your nervous system wants to make life easier for you. It prefers bottom-up processing over top-down processing. Top-down processing—or deliberate action—takes focus and effort, which uses up adrenaline and epinephrine. After a while, effort feels hard and you get tired of doing it. That's why your brain tries to look for patterns to create more and more habits. It tries to move more actions from deliberate to reactionary. Its intention is good—your brain is simply trying to make life easier—but the end result is not so good.

The more your actions become reflexive—almost automatic—the more you are basically sleepwalking through life, not really in control. The only way to make true, lasting change in your life is to take control of your brain, which means taking control of your actions and the thoughts that precede them. This is not a comfortable process, and your brain will fight you on it along the way. It's not because your brain is against you. Your brain is like a computer. It's not emotional—it's simply trying to be more efficient. But efficiency being good for your brain doesn't mean it's good for your life. So when you start breaking patterns and doing new things, it will feel challenging and frustrating. That's just because your brain is now having to think instead of just reacting the way it's always reacted. But here's a Joey quote I want you to remember (maybe write it down somewhere you'll see it often): Stop reacting and start processing. Processing is where change can happen.

WHY DOPAMINE IS SO DOPE

Dopamine is a neurotransmitter, meaning your body uses it to send messages between nerve cells. What most people know about dopamine is that it's associated with the body's reward center. That's why so many people are addicted to social media—they get quick little hits of dopamine with every like or comment their posts get. But dopamine can be used for so much more.

So how do you use this knowledge to your advantage? It's all about creating a journey with rewards along the way so you can get those constant dopamine drips and keep making progress. Don't save your reward for an end, like reaching certain results. Instead, reward yourself throughout the journey.

> Here's a Minimum Method tip about rewards—they do not need to be physical. Get out of the mindset of rewarding yourself with a beer or a sweet treat because you "earned it." That's BS to me. It's time to recognize that rewards can be internal as well.

Let's use working out as an example. Say you want to start going to the gym consistently. The first step in that journey could be buying some new training clothes (or even this book). After you buy the new clothes, take a moment to tell yourself that the clothes are important tools for continuing on your journey to get healthier. Allow yourself to see the purchase as a good thing—a reward—for taking that important step on the journey. The next day, when you go to the gym to sign up for a membership—even if you don't actually train that day—stop and congratulate yourself for taking that next step. Tell yourself you've made a really good move for your overall health and well-being, maybe more than you've ever done before. And when you return to the gym to train (maybe to do a workout from this book), recognize the importance of that step. Are you starting to see a pattern here? The point is to recognize and celebrate every step of the journey.

Notice that I didn't say to reward yourself once you get to where you're working out seven days a week. It's not about the end result—it's always about the journey. Once you do start working out, those rewards will start to become physical, and I'm not just talking about fat loss or muscle gain. Exercise itself will give you a nice hit of dopamine. So it's on you to intentionally get your dopamine hits through internal rewards, then your body will soon join you and double your efforts. You can take this concept and apply it to anything from getting healthier to learning a new language.

Now, using dopamine to your advantage requires intention. You have to be intentional with your thoughts and honest with yourself about how you feel. You see, our brains love patterns and habits, and all our habits are based on feedback loops. When you do something that elicits a positive response (whether it be physical, mental, or emotional), that creates a positive feedback loop, and you're more likely to do it again. And the opposite is true. When you do something with negative consequences, you're less likely to do it again. But here's the kicker—life is all about how we see the world, and we get to choose how we see it. How you choose to see the world is what your brain takes as truth, hence the saying perception is reality.

For example, let's say you have a stressful morning so you decide you're going to eat some comfort food and order a pizza for lunch. By doing that—by telling yourself that pizza is a reward—you're setting an expectation in your brain. Your brain is now expecting the pizza to result in a dopamine hit. But after you eat the pizza, you feel pretty sluggish and gross the rest of the day. That should create a negative feedback loop for your brain because you don't want to feel like that again. Your brain was expecting a dopamine hit but didn't get one. This is known as a reward prediction error.[1] Your brain predicted a reward it didn't get, so you'll be less likely to repeat that behavior. On the other hand, had you eaten the salmon and asparagus you planned to eat for lunch, you would have felt satisfied and energized the rest of the day and gotten that dopamine hit. Plus internally rewarding yourself for choosing to nourish yourself with clean, whole foods means a double dopamine hit!

But the key word there is *should*. This is where you create your own reality because your brain will only register what you allow it to. You have to be in tune with your body and honest with yourself that you feel like crap after eating the pizza in order to create the negative feedback loop. You have to intentionally recognize the negative feedback loop so it sinks into your brain and becomes your reality. If you simply keep telling yourself that you deserve the pizza and it was fun to eat, you will create a positive feedback loop, and you're more likely to start ordering pizza for lunch more often.

However, sometimes you just have a crappy day. When your day sucks, you can't simply decide to think it's been an amazing day and then miraculously it stops sucking. The mind doesn't work that way. In these moments, it's about coming back to the bigger journey and your bigger purpose. You need to attach meaning to the decisions you're making to find those internal rewards. Remember why you want to get healthier. Keep that at the top of your mind and it will help you stay focused on your journey.

So the next time you want to use some crap excuse to be unhealthy, remind yourself that taking that walk or eating clean will make you feel better in the long run. What you do today determines your tomorrow. I want you to be deliberate with your decisions, both in action and thought. Too often, subconscious thoughts take over. Take a moment to proactively focus on your intent and deliberately think about your journey and what you want to achieve.

For an exercise to help you get in tune with how you really feel and identify patterns, go to joeythurman.com/homework.

YOUR BRAIN ON STRESS

Remember that old marketing campaign showing an egg with the caption, "This is your brain," and next to it a cracked egg with the caption, "This is your brain on drugs"? Well, imagine another picture of a scrambled egg with the caption, "And this is your brain on stress." Stress not only wreaks havoc on your body, but it messes up your brain as well. Stress screws with your memory and your mood. It interrupts how brain cells communicate with each other, and it can even kill brain cells altogether. The bottom line is stress is bad for your brain.

Dr. Sue Varma, psychiatrist, NYU professor, on-air contributor to many national TV shows, and author of *Practical Optimism*, has some helpful insight and exercises to combat stress that she shared with me recently:

> People come in to see me for the negative consequences of stress—from work burnout, depression, anxiety, physical complaints to aftermath of trauma, loss, grief, and couples' problems. I can safely say that in most cases, the stressors have been going on for some time because most folks don't go to see a therapist until the other shoe drops, so to speak.

When I work with clients, I want to empower them with tools that can help them not only get through stress in real time, but also prevent future episodes of it. When it comes to depression, for example, each episode of major depression puts you at a higher risk for developing another one. So whether it's everyday stress or a medical illness like major depressive disorder, I take it very seriously (because unmanaged stress can turn into anxiety and depression) and want to nip it in the bud. Unrelenting and unmanageable stress not only wreaks havoc in the mind but the body as well, shortening our life span and putting us at elevated risk for almost every chronic illness out there, from heart disease to stroke to cancer. And as much as I believe in therapy and medication when necessary, there is nothing like having a set of go-to coping techniques. How do I know if therapy for a patient is working? Because they are using what we discussed the other six days a week.

And the key sometimes is knowing your triggers, and being able to anticipate them. But even if stress creeps up on you, it's okay. These are some tools to use. Sometimes the triggers are in the timing—for most of us being hungry, tired, lonely, or sad.

A few quick mental tricks:

Sometimes when we are stressed, we tend to personalize things, make it about us, when it's really not. De-stressing is about making our outlook more in sync with reality. If you're struggling to think positively (and when I say positively, I actually mean accurately), try to reframe the situation and ask yourself: *What's an alternative way for me to look at this?*

Other times, we stress because we think something bad is going to take over our lives when the reality is it might not have much future consequence. Ask yourself: *Will this matter to me five years from now?*

And when you are beating yourself up, ask yourself: *What advice would I give a friend?* We usually are kinder and more reassuring with others. Self-compassion and being kind, gentle, and understanding go a long way.

I also suggest keeping a worry diary. This is for you to write all of your worries, anything you can come up with. And the effects are actually counterintuitive—the more you worry, and write them down, the more you realize most of what you worry about doesn't actually come true. And when it does, you are actually better equipped to handle it than you give yourself credit for.

And finally, to jazz up your mood, ask yourself: *If everything turns out just as I hoped, what would that look like?* When people are worried or anxious, I say, "What's the worst case scenario? What's the best case scenario?" And then I ask, "What is the most likely scenario?"

A few more hacks: I love warm baths, aromatherapy, stretching, power naps, a quick walk, and a comedy show or video. All serve as temporary distractions. However, talking about things, venting to a close friend, or therapy—getting to the root of the issue—will be more helpful in the long run.

Key habits: I call them the four *m*'s of mental health, science-backed behaviors: Every day, get **m**ovement (walk, bike, yoga, etc.), try your hand at **m**astery (do something fun and creative that challenges you just a bit), participate in **m**eaningful engagement (laugh with a friend or connect with a person daily, in person if at all possible), and do something **m**indfully (pay attention to people in your life or try and be present wholeheartedly in whichever activity you are engaged in).

Reducing stress is not about toxic positivity, pretending everything is okay, but, rather, realigning your outlook with reality.

My good friend, famous executive producer, previous podcast guest (season 3, episode 1, *From Rock Bottom to Free Therapy*), and founder of Change Your Algorithm, a free resource for therapy and mental health online, Joel Relampagos also has a couple of quick tricks that can help you de-stress. The first one is to be the MVP! When you wake up in the morning, or whenever you feel stressed, take a couple of minutes to meditate and visualize how you want your day (or the next several hours) to unfold. If negativity arises, shift your perspective. Another trick is to bring your brain out of the current situation by focusing on something else. The next time you're feeling stressed, identify five things you can see, four you can touch, three you can hear, two you can smell, and one you can taste.

FOOD & YOUR MOOD

What we eat has a direct influence on our brain, which is arguably the most important organ we have. Food is so important to our mental health that there is a new field called nutritional psychiatry, where a psychiatrist addresses a person's lifestyle and the food they eat, as well as conduct talk therapy before prescribing medication.

Drew Ramsey, MD, a psychiatrist and author of the book *Eat to Beat Depression and Anxiety*, is a leader in the field of nutritional psychiatry, and I was fortunate to have him as a guest on my podcast (season 3, episode 7, *Food to Fix Depression and Anxiety*). Dr. Ramsey has countless examples of how he's been able to significantly help his patients simply by changing what they eat. We will get into diet in chapter five, but the point I want to make here is that food directly affects our gut, which we now know are our second brain. Our gut is referred to as our second brains because it is linked to the intellectual and emotional brain centers.

Our gut has an enteric nervous system, a vast network of brain-like neurons and neurotransmitters that directly speaks to the brain much like the brain speaks to the rest of the body. In fact we even have gut sensory epithelial cells known as neuropod cells. These neuropod cells provide the base for the gut to send signals to the brain.[2] There's even new research that shows these neuropods can actually dictate a propensity to want sweet foods or not.[3]

Our second brains greatly impact our main brains, a.k.a. the one sitting in your beautiful heads. What's good for our second brain is good for our main brain. And our second brain needs nutrients like iron, potassium, and fatty acids from whole foods to create healthy gut microbiomes, which can then help decrease oxidative stress, reduce inflammation in both the body and the brain, and increase neuroplasticity in the brain.

Your GI tract is lined with hundreds of millions of neurons. As you digest your food, it gets absorbed in your GI tract, then those hundreds of millions of neurons send signals to your brain. What do the signals say? It depends on what you eat. Nutrient-dense healthy whole foods communicate happy signals to your brain, whereas sugary or highly processed foods communicate not-so-happy signals to your brain.

There have been numerous studies comparing the mental health of people who eat a standard American diet (a.k.a. a SAD diet) and those who eat a diet based more in whole foods, like the Mediterranean diet. These studies showed that the people who ate more whole foods had a rate of depression 25 to 35 percent lower than the people who ate a SAD diet, which is known for a lot of highly processed food, refined carbohydrates, added sugars, high-fat dairy, and red meat. These studies show a massive correlation between what we eat and how our brains work in terms of how we perceive the world and regulate our emotions.

A 2017 study named the SMILES (supporting modification of lifestyle in lowered emotional states) Study showed that diet alone—without adding exercise or any other lifestyle modifications—can help improve mood and reduce symptoms of depression.[4] I know that when I don't eat well, I might feel good at the moment, but I'm going to pay for it days later both mentally and physically (no one likes to be bloated). The bottom line is the food we fuel our bodies with plays an incredibly important role in our mental health.

Dr. Ramsey and psychiatrist Dr. Laura LaChance developed the antidepressant food score. Out of thirty-four nutrients, they identified twelve that are key to our mental health and can help prevent and treat depressive disorders.[5] That's right, food alone can help you feel better mentally.

Dr. Ramsey recommends you incorporate the following foods into your day to ensure you're not just eating for your body but for your mind as well.

ANTIDEPRESSANT FOOD SCORE

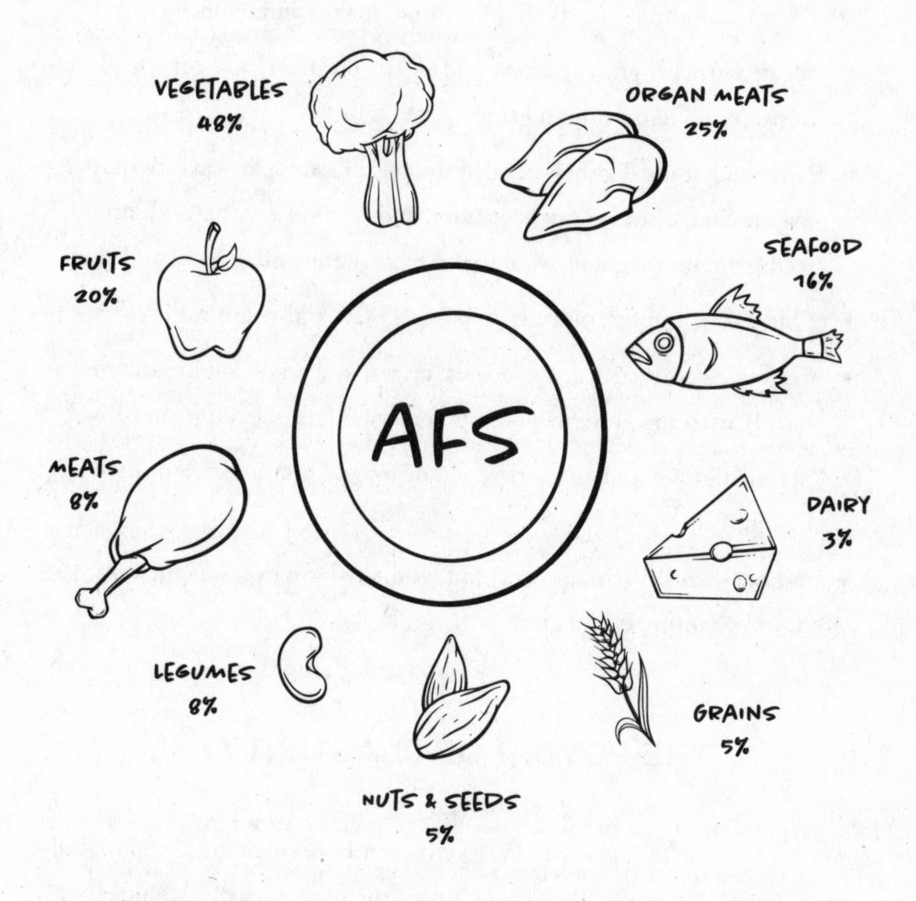

FOOD CATEGORIES & MEAN ANTIDEPRESSANT FOOD SCORE (%)

- Beans: Depending on the type, beans offer an array of thiamine, magnesium, zinc, copper, selenium, manganese, vitamin K, and B vitamins.
- Fermented foods: A lot of research shows how fermented foods like kimchi and pickles, which contain probiotics, can help microbiome diversity and gut health.[6]

- Fruits: Avocados and berries, for example, have B vitamins, magnesium, potassium, and vitamin C.
- Leafy greens: Spinach and kale contain B vitamins, iron, magnesium, zinc, and vitamins A and E.
- Legumes: Lentils have B vitamins, iron, magnesium, and zinc.
- Meat: Go with grass-fed beef and organ meats, which contain B vitamins, iron, vitamin A, and zinc.
- Nuts and seeds: Cashews and walnuts, for example, have B vitamins, magnesium, omega-3 fats, selenium, and vitamin E. Chia and sunflower seeds contain magnesium, omega-3 fats, vitamins B_1 and E, and zinc.
- Oils: Olive and fish oil contain omega-3 fats and vitamin E.
- Seafood: Foods such as anchovies, clams, and wild-caught salmon contain B vitamins, iron, magnesium, omega-3 fats, selenium, and zinc.
- Spices: Ginger and turmeric contain magnesium and vitamins B_1, B_6, C, and E.
- Whole grains: Farro, quinoa, and wild rice have iron, magnesium, selenium, vitamin B_1, and zinc.

THE POWER OF PLASTICITY

Plasticity describes neurons' ability to change their connections and how they work in response to the person's experiences. Greater plasticity helps make it easier for a person to adapt and learn. It is well known that children are information absorbers. We often refer to them as sponges. This is because their young brains have more plasticity, making them more capable of learning and adapting to change. As we grow up, our brains become less plastic; however we are still able to learn and change. But that explains why we become so habitual. For example, we drive the same route to work, sit in the same seat in a conference room, and park in the same general area at the grocery store. These habits and patterns

ANTIDEPRESSANT FOODS

ANTIDEPRESSANT ANIMAL FOODS	AFS RANGE
OYSTER	56%
LIVER & ORGAN MEATS	18-38%
POULTRY GIBLETS	31%
CLAM	30%
MUSSELS	28%
OCTOPUS	27%
CRAB	24%
GOAT	23%
TUNA	15-21%
SMELT	20%
FISH ROE	19%
BLUEFISH	19%
WOLFFISH	19%
POLLOCK	18%
LOBSTER	17%
RAINBOW TROUT	16-17%
SNAIL OR WHELK	16%
SPOT FISH	16%
SALMON	10-16%
HERRING	16%
EMU	16%
SNAPPER	16%

ANTIDEPRESSANT PLANT FOODS	AFS RANGE
WATERCRESS	127%
SPINACH	97%
MUSTARD, TURNIP, BEET GREENS	76-93%
LETTUCES	74-99%
SWISS CHARD	90%
FRESH HERBS	73-75%
CHICORY GREENS	74%
PUMMELO	69%
PEPPERS	39-56%
KALE & COLLARDS	48-62%
PUMPKIN	46%
DANDELION GREENS	43%
CAULIFLOWER	41-42%
KOHLRABI	41%
RED CABBAGE	41%
BROCCOLI	41%
BRUSSELS SPROUTS	35%
ACEROLA	34%
BUTTERNUT SQUASH	34%
PAPAYA	31%
LEMON	31%
STRAWBERRY	31%

aren't inherently bad, but they can become problematic when we aren't aware of them, and we end up "sleepwalking" through life.

When you want to change anything about your life, you have to tap into plasticity. The brain and nervous system are unique in that they change in response to experiences, and luckily keep this ability throughout your entire life span. But to change your brain and your patterns, you have to do something new or push yourself further than you've gone before. And that is something people tend to be resistant to.

Ever notice when you focus for a long time on a new subject, it can leave you feeling agitated? This is the frustration that comes with trying or learning something new, and it's the result of a rush of adrenaline. This agitation is normal, even a good sign. It's your brain getting ready to learn and become more adaptive to plasticity.

Knowing that doesn't necessarily make it less frustrating when you experience it. But here's the thing. Simply becoming aware of those feelings when they happen will help you accept them. And once you get more used to those feelings, your brain can become more plastic. Think of it as growing pains for your brain.

So when it comes to building and maintaining plasticity, novelty is the key. Drive a new way home, try new restaurants, park in a different spot. Maybe don't use your GPS and try to get somewhere without your phone. It's that simple. Take it from my good friend and former podcast guest Sam Effarah, PsyD, BCN, FAIS, founder and CEO of Synapse Chicago (season 1, episode 2, *Brain Training*), who says:

> Over the past twenty-five years I have devoted my life to being a student of the human brain. I have learned that the brain is like a finely tuned engine. It consumes a great deal of energy and is also subject to wear and tear as it ages. If you want your brain to perform at its maximum potential for years to come, one important key is novelty.
>
> What does novelty mean in regards to the brain? Challenge the brain to acquire new skills in a variety of areas so that positive neural pathways are enriched. This allows your brain to be more flexible, which results in optimal performance and cognition.

- Practice a new instrument.
- Learn a new language.
- Take a class in an academic subject that you do not understand.
- Change up your training routine.

Novelties like these are like the oil in the engine. They keep the brain functioning at its peak as it strengthens all the regions, so they work together optimally and efficiently as you age.

As time goes on and we become more aware that the frustration that comes with trying something new means growth, our brains will begin to associate the discomfort with a reward instead of fear and agitation. That's when real change happens.

WHEN YOU CHANGE YOUR BRAIN, YOU CHANGE YOUR LIFE

It is easier to become more plastic from birth through about age twenty-five, but that doesn't mean you're out of luck if you've already celebrated your twenty-fifth birthday. You can self-direct your plasticity. You are in charge. It's as simple as deciding to change. Okay, simple . . . but not always easy. Understanding this can help you better understand yourself and how you can change. If you want to change yourself, you need to stop and think about what exactly you are trying to change, whether it's your perceptions, emotions, thoughts, or behaviors. Then determine the path needed to make the change happen.

All change starts in the brain and you can in fact decide to change your brain. Jeffrey Schwartz, MD, is a neuropsychiatrist and author of several books, including *Brain Lock: Free Yourself from Obsessive-Compulsive Disorder.* He works with all sorts of people but specializes in those with obsessive-compulsive disorder (OCD). He doesn't prescribe these patients pills to overcome their OCD, but he gets them to work on a four-step process to actively change their behavior. The process includes four *r*'s: relabel, reattribute, refocus, and revalue. While I'm sure that not everyone reading this has OCD, the process is really valuable to help with any kind of change.

- Relabel: This addresses our brain glitches, or false messages. A false message could be anything from thinking that you have to check your phone first thing in the morning to thinking that if you can't train for a full hour, it isn't worth it. Relabeling involves recognizing those thoughts and changing them to something like, "It's okay. I know this is just my pattern of behavior to check my phone, but work, social media, and texts will still be there in an hour" or, "Even though I don't have time for a full-hour training session, I can still get twenty minutes in, and doing something is better than doing nothing."

- Reattribute: This is asking yourself why certain thoughts keep coming back. For the phone example, you can simply think, "Oh this is my brain sending messages that I need to check my phone because I'm so used to it but it's a false message." Or for the training example, reattributing is reminding yourself that an hour is a false, arbitrary rule when it comes to exercise. Understanding why you think or do certain things or where they come from can help you with the next step.
- Refocus: This is the hardest step and can be the most frustrating because it's actually changing the behavior. You need to constantly remind yourself of the why associated with the old behavior and then take action to complete a new behavior. This may be turning your phone over, getting up, and starting your new morning routine with some sunlight before ever looking at that phone. After a while of consciously changing the behavior, your brain will change, and the old pattern will be replaced with the new good behavior.
- Revalue: This is the sum of all the three previous steps. You now see your old behavior as something that was distracting to you and didn't add value. The new behavior adds value to your life and you feel better for it. Before you know it, you will think of that old behavior and say, "Why did I ever do that? It did not enhance my life, it only hindered it." From there you can use the four *r*'s to change other behaviors that aren't conducive to your success.

PLAY GAMES

So, time for some minimums to help upgrade your brain. Don't worry, you don't need to get your brain mapped and attached to all sorts of sensors as I have to do for my podcast. It's as simple as playing a game! That's right. The simple act of playing a game of cards or doing a puzzle has been shown to develop cognition and help the brain fight against aging. Even one quick game of cards can lead to more volume in regions of the brain! So the next time you feel like you need to work your brain muscle, simply reach for a game you loved as a kid and grab someone to play with you.

Games that help maintain your cognition include computer games, crafting, and social activities. A study published in *Neurology* found a 20 percent reduction in mild cognitive impairment when people middle aged or older engaged in social activities like playing games with friends or even going to the movies.[7] Although this study was observational, meaning self-reported, it still shows a strong correlation with being social and stimulating the mind.

Studies also suggest that doing puzzles can keep your mind sharp as you age. A study published in the *International Journal of Geriatric Psychiatry* showed that word puzzles, crossword puzzles, and number puzzles like sudoku can keep the brain working longer for people fifty years and older.[8] A 2017 study published in *Neurology* followed 1,903 people well into their eighties for seven years and found that those who engaged in reading, board games, cards, and puzzles had a delayed onset of dementia by up to five years.[9] These studies show that playing games and interacting in a social setting seem to be the key to keeping our brains young and healthy.

Here's a Minimum Method tip when playing games—play with family or friends. Surrounding yourself with loved ones is one of the best things you can do for brain health. Every part of our souls wants to feel loved and connected, and it turns out that our brains need that, too.

The brain also needs to be constantly challenged and engaged, so it's not enough to keep doing the same games or puzzles. You will simply just get better at those activities. Instead, try to keep making your activity more difficult. My son and father-in-law, Dean, are like best friends, and they love to do puzzles together. Rather than do the same puzzle over again, Dean makes it harder by turning the puzzle pieces over, forcing him and Frederic to complete the puzzle using only the shapes and no colors to guide them. The new layer of difficulty creates a little stress, which we've discussed is good because it helps brains stay more plastic and open to change and new information. The key—even with games—is to change your routine to keep your brain from plateauing.

Here's a list of games I recommend for brain health:

- Crossword puzzles: Pick up almost any newspaper—if you can even find an actual newspaper—and chances are there will be a crossword puzzle inside. You can also search online for crossword puzzles and set difficulty levels. Remember (pun intended), that making your brain work harder is good, so make sure to bump up the intensity level as the puzzles get easier. Crossword puzzles also help increase vocabulary, which not only makes you sound smart, but also helps with memory recall when you are in a conversation. When you find a new word, look it up and try to integrate it into a sentence that day.
- Sudoku: Sudoku is a game that uses a grid and numbers. But don't worry. There isn't that much math involved. It helps you increase your logic and working memory. You can find these puzzles in apps, books, and all over the web. The *New York Times* releases Sudoku puzzles in different difficulty levels from easy to hard every day on its website.
- Jigsaw puzzles: Jigsaw puzzles are a great way to use the right side of your brain, which is thought to be the creative side, as well as the more logical left side of the brain. Solving a jigsaw puzzle involves visuospatial functioning, provides a nice parasympathetic calming response, and can be done with friends.

- Scrabble: I've never been much of a Scrabble player, but my wife kicks my ass every time we play. On top of increasing your vocabulary and forcing you to recollect vocabulary you often wouldn't use, Scrabble also has a puzzle component and requires strategy and logical thinking.
- Simon Says: Remember this one from childhood? Simon Says forces you to use deliberate focus while listening for the words *Simon Says*. Deliberately focusing attention on someone's words as well as directing that attention to action can increase awareness and balance. It's also a fun game and will help you laugh more.

> Laughter is key for overall health because it stimulates many organs (including the brain), helps the stress response, soothes tension, increases the immune system by releasing neuropeptides that help fight stress and illness, and improves mood and depressive symptoms.[10]

The value in playing games is much more than simply the game part. It's the social interaction—playing games with friends—that makes games extra beneficial. Too often as people age, they spend less time socializing with friends, and it is those personal connections that can help someone age better and live longer. In neuroscientist Daniel Levitin's book, *Successful Aging*, he talks about the importance of keeping a strong social circle, especially as we age, for proper brain development.

TUNE IN

One of the easiest ways to help your brain is to listen to music. Not just any music, though. When it comes to brain health, Mozart really was onto something. In 1991, it was hypothesized that listening to Mozart's music could make children smarter.[11] This eventually became known as the Mozart effect. But interestingly enough, when you look at the original paper, the study was done on young adults, not children.

Here's what the Mozart experiment showed. College students were asked to look at folded pieces of paper and make an educated guess as to what the pieces would look like unfolded. The group that listened to Mozart performed better than the group that did not. But the "extra smarts" only lasted for about fifteen minutes. Years later, a meta-analysis of sixteen different studies confirmed that music does lead to a temporary improvement in the ability to mentally manipulate shapes.[12] *Temporary* being the operative word.

Other studies have looked at different types of music besides Mozart and found that listening to Schubert or even a passage from a novel helped learning capabilities, but only if the person enjoyed it. Furthermore, listening to Mozart has been shown (in rats) to increase the gene expression of brain-derived neurotrophic factor (BDNF), a neural growth factor; cAMP response element binding protein (CREB),[13] a compound for learning and memory; and synapse, a synaptic growth protein. In other words "smart" brain chemicals are stimulated by music.

So is it the type of music or the mere enjoyment of it that matters? A 2006 study of eight thousand children found they experienced cognitive arousal while listening to music in general, no matter if it was classical or pop. So the conclusion here is that music is good for the brain, but you have to enjoy it. Besides the enjoyment factor, music is also relaxing and promotes the ability to focus more by reducing mental and physical stress in the moment and by turning on that parasympathetic nervous system (PNS) state.

Find music that makes you feel good and doesn't stress you out. For example, I'm not going to listen to my heavy metal workout music while trying to write this book. That pumps me up for a training session, but for writing I need calming classical music. Find music that works for whatever task you're doing and put it on in the background. If you are doing certain tasks that require more special memory, or if you are going to take a test, listen to some music beforehand for better cognition.

THE ART OF DOING NOTHING

When was the last time you did nothing? I really mean it, nothing at all. What does nothing mean? Well, put your phone down, turn off the television, shut out any outside noise, and simply just be with yourself. In a minute, I want you to put this book down and do just that. I want you to simply close your eyes and let your mind wonder. Pay attention to what sounds you hear. Think about what you're grateful for. Notice how your body feels. Do you feel wind on your face? Do you feel relaxed or tense? Then after a couple of minutes, you can open your eyes and resume reading. Okay, go!

Welcome back and congratulations—you just meditated! Yes, I know. You thought you had to be on top of a mountain somewhere enchanting surrounded by monks or have some bearded guru in front of you. Nope. Mediation and the art of doing nothing has a lot of positive benefits. Simply taking a few minutes for yourself every day and doing nothing has been shown to lessen feelings of depression and anxiety, help with IBS, and a lot more. So the next time you have nothing to do, I want you to think about what that nothing can do for you!

Doing nothing doesn't have to be meditation. *Non-sleep deep rest* is a term coined by Dr. Andrew Huberman, who was a guest on my podcast (season 2, episode 7, *Optimizing Your Life, Brain, and Day*). He talks about the importance of doing things that rest your body and help your mind. Some examples include breathing exercises (more on this later), meditation, self-reflection, and, one of my favorites, yoga nidra, a guided meditative state between waking and sleeping.

> Here's a Minimum Method tip. Yoga nidra is one of the simplest things you can do to calm yourself and your nervous system down. Simply google *yoga nidra,* click on a video, and listen to the cues and lovely sounds to calm you down. You can do this in the morning, afternoon, or evening. Do this as often as you'd like. No need for fancy meditation techniques.

BRING IN BRAIN SUPPORT

Now, you may be thinking, "Okay, Joey. Games sound fun, and I can certainly do nothing, but is there anything I can do to help my brain act like a happy, fast-learning kid again?" Why, yes there is.

As you know, this book is about the little things. We don't always need big changes to reach big results. When it comes to brain health, several supplements have shown promise of getting your quick wit back and even preventing Alzheimer's.

Nootropics are a classification of supplements that can enhance your mental cognition and learning, support verbal recall, and more. Here are my favorite nootropics:

- *Bacopa monnieri*: *Bacopa monnieri* is an herb used for centuries in ayurvedic medicine that has been found to increase the length and branching of nerve cells. Translation: This helps your memory. The herb also helps with oxidative stress and prevents cognitive decline.
- Phosphatidylserine: Phosphatidylserine is a nutrient found in the cerebral cortex that helps carry messages between cells. Again, this helps your memory.
- Caffeine with theanine: Theanine is an amino acid that can relax you but not make you sleepy or fatigued. Taken with caffeine, it acts synergistically to reduce the over excitability of caffeine and increase your focus and attention span. Take 200 milligrams of theanine with a 200-milligram caffeine tablet, one to three cups of coffee depending on strength. If you are not used to caffeine, take 50 milligrams of each. If taken on an empty stomach, it can increase the absorption rate but may give you stomach issues. If you no longer feel the effects of caffeine, slowly cycle off for two weeks and then go back on.
- Blueberries: What? I know, blueberries aren't typically considered a supplement, but this tiny, delicious little berry should be a core food and supplement in your arsenal. I eat about three pounds per week, no joke.

Talk about fruit fuel! Anthocyanins and pterostilbene in blueberries have been shown to protect the brain and reduce cognitive decline.[14] There is also evidence of improved episodic memory, executive function, and working memory. Try to take one of the following every day: 12 grams of blueberry powder, ¼ cup (24 grams) of freeze-dried sugar-free blueberries, 60 to 120 grams of fresh or frozen blueberries, or two cups (170 ounces) of pure blueberry juice (sugar-free).

Another option is to eat more mushrooms. That's right, mushrooms. But not the shrooms you're used to seeing in the grocery store. There are so many different types of mushrooms, and many of them help with brain health, energy, and cognition. For example, reishi stimulates nerve cell growth in the brain and protects against seizures, and lion's mane has tremendous brain health properties and antioxidant benefits, and can give your whole body more energy. You can find these mushrooms and more in supplement form. I often take my shrooms in my morning coffee and add in a little cocoa powder—it's delicious!

THE MINIMUM METHOD BRAIN PROTOCOLS

Let's Go!

- Use dopamine to your advantage by identifying and celebrating small wins along your health journey.
- Pay attention to how you feel both mentally and physically after making certain decisions, such as what you eat and how you spend your time. What makes you feel good and energized, and what makes you feel down and sluggish? Be honest with yourself and start to identify patterns to build and reinforce positive feedback loops.
- Incorporate stress management strategies, whether it be keeping a worry diary, venting to a friend, or going to therapy.
- Work on brain plasticity by switching up some of your routines, such as the route you drive to work and where you park at the grocery store.

Level Up!

- Incorporate the four *m*'s of mental health daily—movement, mastery, meaningful engagement, and mindfulness.
- Incorporate foods from Dr. Ramsey's list that help with mental health.
- Play classical music in the background while you work or study.
- Work on brain plasticity by trying to learn something new, like a language or an instrument.
- Do some form of meditation every day, even if it's simply sitting and doing nothing but breathing.

Max Out!

- Start your day with MVP—meditate, visualize your day, and put things into perspective.
- Start taking some of the brain support supplements listed in the chapter.
- Incorporate more games into your life, ideally with family or friends.

4

BREATHWORK IS THE BEST WORK

Right now, at this moment, are you thinking about your breathing? You probably are now that I mentioned it, but most of the time, we breathe without thinking or even noticing it. It's automatic. Turns out, there is a lot of power in this seemingly simple bodily function. It has shown to help with training, recovery, stress, and more. Even the involuntary yawn has its purpose. Yawning helps bring more oxygen into the blood and then move carbon dioxide out of the blood.

BREATHING 101: YOU'RE DOING IT WRONG

You may be wondering why I've included an entire chapter on breathing, something you've done your entire life without even thinking about it. And yes, you are partly correct. Breathing is something we supposedly do automatically, like walking, running, and chewing. We do these perfectly and rarely give them a second thought, that is until someone points out how and why to do them correctly. I implore you to read this chapter and practice breathing correctly. This could be one of the best things you ever do for your health.

The breath is thought to be directly linked to the autonomic nervous system, which includes the parasympathetic nervous system, sympathetic nervous system, and enteric nervous system. We now know that if we consciously think about what we do and how we breathe, we can have a direct effect on the nervous system, impacting heart rate, stress levels, digestive processes, and a lot more. So as you read the words on this page, I want you to focus on your breath. Are you breathing through your nose or your mouth? Do you feel like you are getting enough air? Are you fully exhaling and inhaling, or are your breaths short? I know—it's a lot that you likely haven't paid much attention to in your life. But how you breathe can be linked to every cell in your body. Breathing directly affects recovery, metabolic rate, the ability to fight off pathogens, and sleep, just to name a few things.

Babies breathe strictly through their noses, which is called obligate nose breathing. The only time babies breathe through their mouths is when they're crying. The reason for this is that babies don't have any cartilage in their noses when they are born so the nasal passages are wide open. That's also why babies shouldn't sleep on their stomachs—when their noses get pressed down, there is no cartilage to keep the air passages open. As we grow up and get older, we start to breathe through our mouths more, which is not beneficial for us. Breathing through the mouth is meant to be a backup in case of congestion or needing air quickly, but it has become common. We've become a bunch of mouth breathers.

In this chapter, I'm going to give you a number of tools to help you breathe better overall and use breathing to train better, sleep better, de-stress, and even heighten alertness when needed. But first, let's start with just trying to breathe normally.

It is estimated that only 25 to 50 percent of the world's population breathes through their noses. And from what I've seen, I wouldn't be surprised if that number was low. Breathing through our noses warms the air, pressurizes it, and cleans it by filtering out junk like allergens. This process allows the lungs to extract oxygen more efficiently. When we exhale through our nostrils, it takes longer and allows us to use oxygen better, as exhalation increases our absorption rate of oxygen. When we breathe through our mouths, we get none of these benefits.

Scientists have known this for a long time, but it wasn't known just how detrimental not breathing properly was until much more recently with the release of James Nestor's book *Breath*. He scoured the planet to figure out why we breathe and how to breathe properly. He even did a crazy experiment with Stanford scientist Dr. Jayakar Nayak, where he first blocked his nostrils for ten days, forcing him to breathe solely through his mouth, and then he released his nostrils and taped his mouth shut for ten days to solely breathe through his nose.

What happened was incredible! Within one day of only mouth breathing, Nestor's snoring increased by 1,000 percent, he developed sleep apnea, his blood pressure increased by 15 percent, his heart rate variability (HRV) went to shit, and he had a lot more issues. Can you imagine how bad things would have gotten for him if this experiment had continued for longer than ten days? Then when he switched to only nose breathing, his snoring, sleep apnea, and all other symptoms went away. This is only one example but still highly enlightening. Think of the health issues that could be solved by simply breathing correctly. We've gotten to the point where people are using machines so they can breathe at night when the simple fix could be to just stop mouth breathing and start breathing out of your nose like we were designed to.

If that hasn't convinced you to breathe through your nose, consider the discovery from Nobel Prize winner Dr. Louis Ignarro, who codiscovered the gas nitric oxide (NO) and how important it is to us. When you breathe through your nose into your lungs, the air has a high concentration of NO, but it is not present when you breathe through your mouth. That's because NO is made by the nasal mucosal cells within the nose. NO is a smooth-muscle relaxing agent, so when you breathe it in, it relaxes the tracheal smooth muscles and bronchial muscles, widening them and allowing in more air. It also helps with pulmonary circulation by dilating the small pulmonary arteries and capillaries so they can get more blood in the lungs, which in turn pick up more oxygen. The oxygenated blood is then carried to the rest of the body. NO is antimicrobial as well. It's a reactive free radical and can kill certain microbes, bacteria, parasites, and viruses . . . yes even coronaviruses! It prevents microbes from multiplying and protects us from a lot of the crap in the air.

THE RIGHT WAY TO BREATHE

So before we get into some crazy breathing exercises and techniques (those are coming), let's talk about how to breathe correctly. Be aware that this is going to feel strange and possibly difficult at first because you've probably been a crap breather for years. Don't worry, you're not alone! And remember what we talked about in the brain chapter—agitation is good. So when you feel agitated while working on your breathing, recognize and move toward it, attaching a reward to it.

You are going to focus on lifting your diaphragm as you breathe in and letting it sink down as you exhale. This will help you get 20 percent more oxygen. That's right, 20 percent more! Because breathing with your diaphragm helps bring more blood to the thoracic cavity and pushes it through the heart, almost like a second pump. Most likely you are a chest breather and not properly breathing through your diaphragm. So here's how to do it correctly.

First, place one hand on your chest and one hand on your stomach above your belly button. Then give yourself a full exhale out of your nose. Now take a deep breath in through your nose and feel your stomach expand. Breathe through your hand on your stomach so that your stomach extends out during the first two-thirds of your breath and then feel your chest open up and ribs expand for the final one-third of the breath. For every breath you take, simply focus on your hand expanding and then your chest. Then focus on your exhale being longer than your inhale. No need to count, just focus on the exhale being at least a little bit longer than your inhale. You want to fully exhale so you get all the old air out.

Breathing like that is something all of us can do. Start by practicing it while you aren't doing anything and then you can move on to trying it during your daily life, like while you're taking a walk or even walking up stairs. It will take a few weeks to get used to breathing like this, but doing so will help with snoring and sleep apnea, and you will sleep better overall. Once you master breathing during the day, it's time to try some mouth tape at night. (If you feel like you're having a bigger breathing problem, I suggest you see a breathing specialist.)

CHECK YOUR BREATH

By checking your breath, I don't mean breathing into your hand to see if your breath smells. It's time to check the quality of your breathing.

In the 1950s, Russian doctor Konstantin Buteyko developed a way to test breathing quality called control pause (CP). His method has been proven to help with overbreathing, which causes excess oxygen consumption, too much carbon dioxide exhalation, and—you guessed it—usually mouth breathing. Dr. Buteyko found that people should actually be breathing less, making only a "whisper" in and out of their noses as they breathe. So basically, not only are we breathing incorrectly, but we are also overbreathing! Using the CP method can help increase NO as well as maintain healthy carbon dioxide levels, which helps with heart function and much more. I'll give you a quick rundown of the CP technique, but for more specific instructions and information, go to buteykoclinic.com.

When you do the CP test, it's important to be in a calm state, meaning you didn't just train or have an argument with someone. The most accurate time to do it is first thing in the morning. Basically, what you're going to do is inhale calmly through your nose, then exhale. At the end of your exhale, pinch your nostrils closed so you can't inhale again. You want to time how long it takes until you feel that first urge to inhale, called air hunger. That part is important. You aren't timing how long you can hold your breath. You're timing how long it takes until you feel the urge breathe. When you inhale again, it shouldn't be

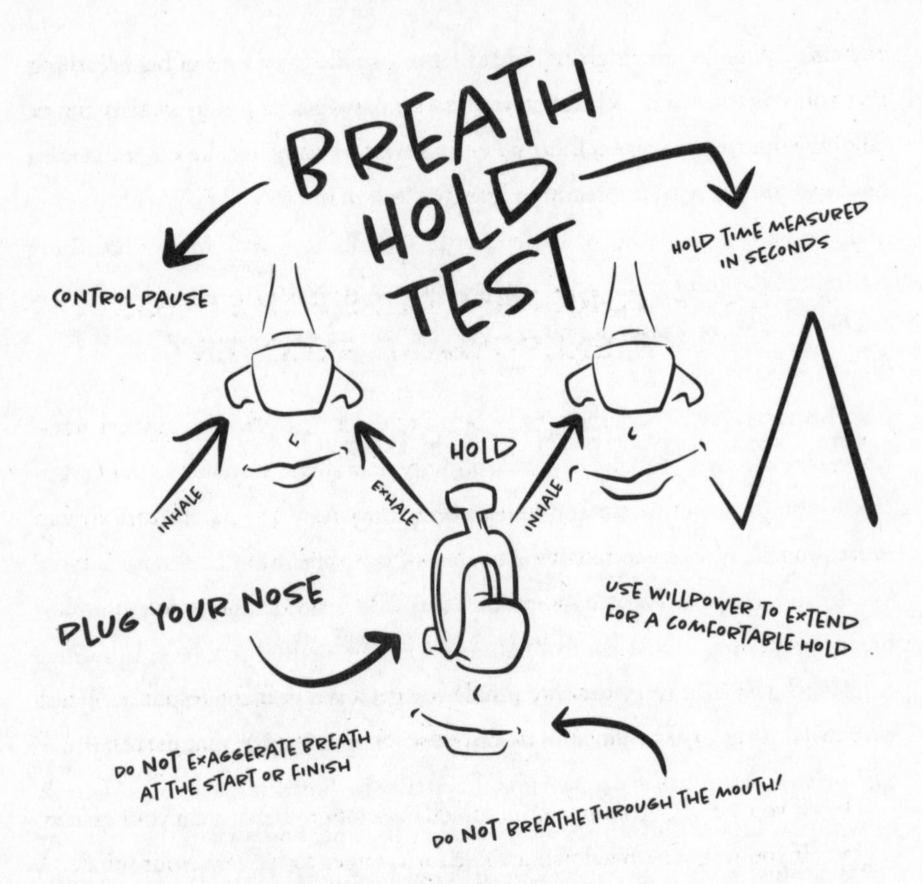

labored at all. It should be as calm as before you pinched your nostrils closed. If you have to take a big inhale or it is labored at all, you went past the point of air hunger.

Your goal is to reach a CP of forty seconds. Don't freak out if yours is much lower. The first time I did it, I got twenty-three seconds. Your score is an indication of your breathing volume. The lower your score, the higher volume breather you are. High volume breathers are more prone to stress and anxiety than people with a high CP. So how do you increase your CP? Well, basically, do what I talk about in this book—breathe through your nose, still your mind (hello meditation!), and exercise. You need to become more aware of your breathing throughout the day and try to avoid "big breathing." Your breath should be quiet and calm. And no more sighing. That's right—sighing is a type of big breathing that you want to avoid. When you feel the urge to sigh, stop it by swallowing or holding your breath. Again, there's a lot more information on the CP method so head over to the Buteyko Clinic website to check it out.

BREATHWORK PRACTICES FOR STRESS RELIEF, ENERGY, AND RECOVERY

Can we control what was thought to be automatic? Yes! And I'm not just referring to breathing. For a long time, the autonomic nervous system was thought to be without control, involuntary, or unconscious, but we have found that we can in fact control it. I vote to rename it to the responsive system. This name is more fitting because as we become more conscious of this system, our bodies respond to that awareness.

Check this out: every time we inhale, we get a sympathetic response. When we exhale, we get a parasympathetic response. So this is what that means:

- If you want to get amped up, inhale for a longer count than your exhale.
- If you want to slow down, exhale for a longer count than your inhale.
- For balance, inhale for five to six seconds then exhale for five to six seconds.

Knowing these minimum facts can help you gain control over your newfound responsive system. You'll be able to take control of your nervous system and many immune functions with only your breathing.

Before we get into the techniques themselves, a quick note on how to monitor your progress. A great and inexpensive way to see if your breathwork is helping is to get a blood pressure cuff and regularly check your blood pressure to see if your levels improve over time. If you snore, try using an app (I like Snorelab) that measures your snoring so you can see what improves it, whether it is a breathing strip, doing breathing exercises before bed, or using mouth tape.

BREATHING THROUGH STRESS

Our breath has the power to move us out of stress mode and into a sense of calm. That's where the saying "just take a deep breath" comes from. When we are stressed, our sympathetic nervous system is activated, and we go into fight-or-flight mode. This is a primal survival response that used to help us run from saber-toothed tigers. It's quite efficient, too. All the blood and energy in our body move away from their regular jobs to essential functions only. Heart rate increases, pupils dilate, and digestion even slows. It's great for lifesaving escapes; not so great for overall long-lasting health.

Taking a deep breath creates a parasympathetic response that counteracts the fight-or-flight mode. It triggers relaxation and allows the body to go back to taking care of itself. Heart rate drops, digestion returns to normal, and we can settle into a sense of calm (which, believe it or not, is supposed to be our natural state). The point is that breath has power.

In the past, every time I thought of breathing exercises, I couldn't help but picture myself sitting in a circle, talking about my emotions, and eating granola. Maybe that's your cup of tea and maybe it isn't. Regardless, we can actually use our breathing patterns consciously in the exact moment we feel stress or need to calm down. This is an incredible tool that can be used in all areas of life. It's no secret that stress isn't good for your health. Breathing is the minimal effort tool for maximum results.

During my podcast interview with Dr. Andrew Huberman, he shared a simple, yet innovative, breathing technique called physiological sighs, initially discovered in the 1930s. In 2016, Dr. Jack Feldman of UCLA and his team discovered how sighing can lead to rapid calming.

Try this between sets the next time you're training or during a stressful event: Inhale deeply through your nose. Without exhaling, inhale again through your nose. Then exhale. Repeat this a few times. This technique allows you to take in twice the oxygen, which improves your heart rate variability and calms

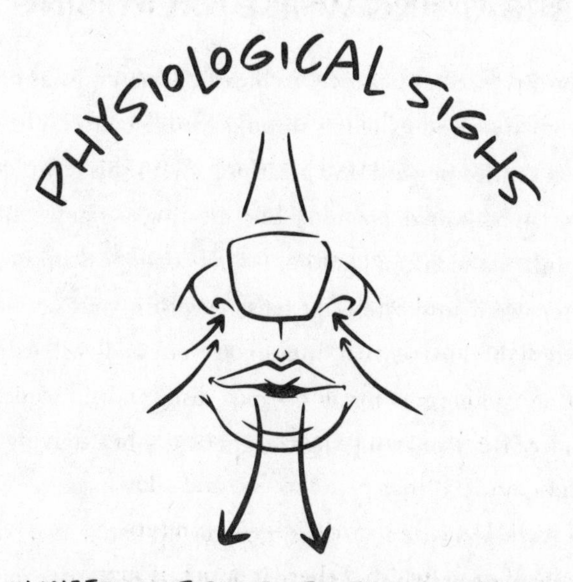

INHALE THROUGH THE NOSE. WITHOUT EXHALING, TAKE AN EXTRA INHALATION THROUGH THE NOSE. THEN, EXHALE, AND REPEAT.

you down faster. It's an excellent hack when training so you can recover faster between sets, get more oxygen, and therefore have a more efficient workout. In fact, it is the fastest way to bring the mind and body into a more relaxed state. Doing one to three of these double inhales will quickly bring your nervous system back to its baseline.

Another breathing technique that has proven to reduce stress is alternate nostril breathing. Close your right nostril with your finger and inhale slowly through your left nostril. Then close your left nostril and exhale slowly through the right nostril. With your left nostril still closed, inhale slowly through your right nostril, then close the right nostril and exhale slowly through the left nostril. Repeat this process for as long as you want. It will help restore balance to your body and nervous system, help you sleep, and much more.[1] Fun fact—we naturally switch which nostril is dominant about every two hours.

BREATHING WHILE EXERCISING

When doing cardio-based exercise, try to breathe as naturally as possible, inhaling through your nose and exhaling through your mouth. When lifting, you want to do what's called power HISS breathing. With this technique, you focus on creating intra-abdominal pressure, like creating a rigid corset to protect your spine. Think of a soda can (and no, I don't condone drinking soda) as you breathe out. You want to create mild tension within your core through your expansion because this load tension throughout your body will help protect your spine by limiting compressive forces on your disks and subsequently help you lift more. Think of this like an internal weight belt or brace giving extra support to your structure.

Have you ever watched a powerlifter do a big lift and notice how their stomach expands? They're creating that tension. So whether you are squatting, pressing, or doing most any other exercise, you want to inhale right before the lift and fill your "soda can," then do the eccentric (the negative or lowering phase) and drive through the concentric, exhaling through the sticking point. So for a push-up, you would breathe in before the movement, lower yourself, then as you start pushing up, exhale once you get to that sticking, or hardest, point.

The key to this technique is that you're matching your breath to the movement in a way that helps with production because you're exhaling through the hardest part. You can practice this while lying on the floor on your back. Place one hand on your stomach above the belly button and the other on your chest. Inhale and practice breathing into your belly so that it, not your chest, rises.

When you're finished exercising, it's time for some recovery breathing. When you train, your body uses more oxygen and produces more carbon dioxide than normal. To handle this increased demand, your breathing will increase from fifteen times per minute at rest to forty to sixty times per minute while exercising.[2] So it's important to down-regulate your system and get back to a parasympathetic state.

To recover, lie on your back with your feet up on a wall or bench at about a 90 degree bend in your knees. Breathe in through your nose for a count of four seconds, hold it at the top for a second or two, then exhale for a count of eight seconds. What matters most here is the 1:2 ratio of inhale to exhale time so you don't need to worry so much about sticking to four- and eight-second counts. Repeat this for a few minutes, and your body will move back into its rest and digest mode.

BREATHING AS AN ENERGY BOOST

Breathwork can also help boost our energy. By providing our cells with more oxygen, they can better fuel our brains and bodies. One breathing technique that is arguably better than coffee is bellows breath. This technique utilizes rapid and forceful breathing that stimulates the diaphragm and makes you more alert, energized, and clear minded. Do this before a training session or anytime you want to focus.

To do it, sit tall with relaxed shoulders. Keep your mouth closed and inhale rapidly through your nose and exhale rapidly through your nose in quick bursts, breathing in and out as your chest elevates and drops with each breath. Start with ten-second rounds, take a fifteen- to thirty-second break, then repeat. Do this several times, and you'll feel like you just had a shot of espresso!

BREATHING TO CALM DOWN

We often try to quiet our minds with our minds, which is counterintuitive. Think about it—if you keep telling your mind to calm down, then you are focusing on how your mind is not quiet and therefore stressing yourself more. Whether it be to fall asleep or simply relax, breathing is a great way to calm down. Here are several breathing techniques that will help quiet your mind and body:

- Box breathing has been incredibly popular over the past several years because it's a great way to calm the mind and system without overthinking. All you have to do is imagine drawing a box with your breath. Simply close your mouth and slowly inhale through your nose for a count of four, then hold your breath for four, exhale through your mouth for four, and hold the exhalation for four. Do this for several rounds.

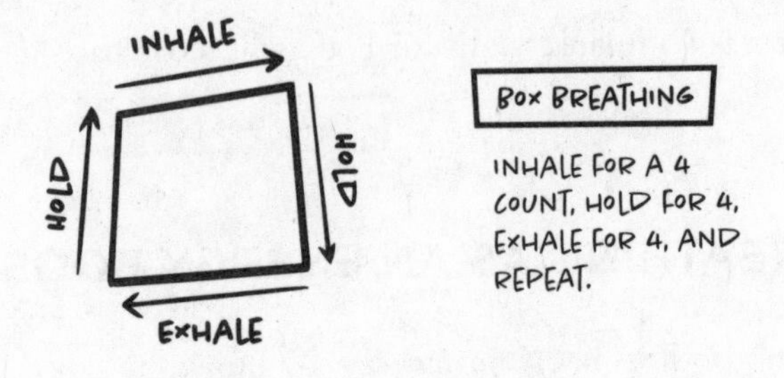

- The 4-7-8 breathing technique is similar in concept to box breathing and one I personally use when I'm lying in bed at night listening to some calming sounds. Place your tongue against the top of your mouth and inhale through your nose for a count of four, hold for a count of seven, and then exhale either through your mouth or nose for a count of eight. Repeat for several rounds.

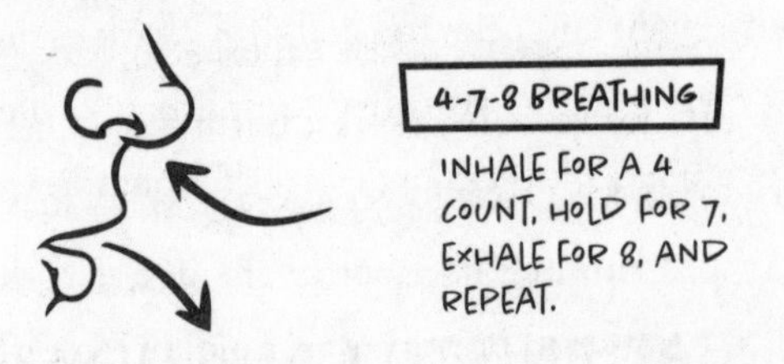

- Five finger breathing brings touch and breath together in one. The simple sensation of touch can also have a calming effect. Take one hand and place it in front of you with your palm facing you. You're going to use the pointer finger from your other hand to trace the hand that's out. Start along the outside of the pinky finger. Slowly inhale as you trace up your finger, pause as you reach the top of the finger, and exhale as you trace down the inside of the finger. Once you reach the web in between your fingers, inhale slowly and repeat the process for all five fingers. Another way to do this is to have someone else trace your finger as you focus on your breathing. It's an amazing way to connect with yourself and with someone else.

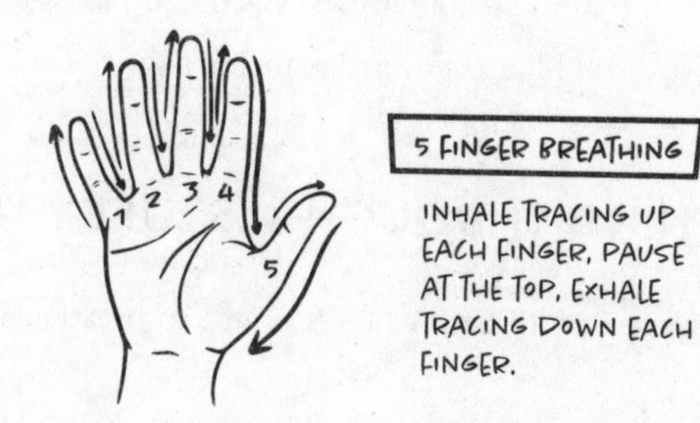

BREATHING FOR OUR IMMUNE SYSTEM

It was once thought that we could not trigger our autonomic nervous system and innate immune system, but practicing the Wim Hof Method (a form of Tummo breathing) can trigger these systems to fight off infection, increase immune function, and even produce anti-inflammatory mediators to down-regulate the pro-inflammatory cytokine response when exposed to bacteria. This breathing technique has been used for years by monks, but it was Wim Hof who made it popular. Don't worry, you don't have to get as crazy as he does, dunking himself in freezing ice baths and running barefoot in the desert without any water, to reap the benefits of this powerful breathing technique. Here's how to do it:

1. Get comfortable in a meditation posture or lying down, allowing your lungs to be open.
2. Close your eyes and try to be calm. Inhale deeply through your nose and exhale without force out of your mouth. Inhale from the belly first and then into the chest. Do this with powerful breaths—but not forced—thirty to forty times. Some people may feel limb tingling or get lightheaded, but this is normal.
3. After the last breath, inhale deeply one more time, then exhale all the air out and hold this as long as you can until you have to take another breath.

4. When you need to breathe, inhale deeply through your belly into your chest, hold it for fifteen seconds, and then let it go.
5. Repeat this for three to four times. According to Wim Hof, this is a perfect way to feel bliss and practice meditation.

BREATHING THROUGH A STUFFY NOSE

You can even use breathing to help when it's hard to breathe. Do this to clear your sinuses:

1. Tilt your head back.
2. Pinch your nose shut.
3. Hold your breath as long as you can.
4. When you exhale, return your head to neutral (look out for the snot), and your sinuses should be clear.

Why does this work? Your brain senses less oxygen and in turn kicks in your survival mechanism to get more oxygen, and it clears your sinuses.

Do this to clear a stuffy nose:

1. Exhale calmly.
2. Pinch your nose shut.
3. Nod up and down a few times, then move your head from side to side a few times.
4. Hold your breath as long as you can.
5. When you need to breathe, slowly breathe through your nose.
6. Repeat until you are able to breathe easily through your nose.

TIME TO STOP SNORING

If you snore, it's because as you are sleeping, the space behind your tongue narrows and the tissue around it becomes relaxed and floppy. Air tries to get through this small passage, which causes the tissue to flutter, and this vibration produces a lovely snoring melody. When you have sleep apnea, the floppy muscles in the back of your throat relax so much that they completely close off your airway and that's not good. This decreases how much oxygen you're getting and disrupts your sleep.

But does snoring always mean you have sleep apnea? Unfortunately, most likely. Snoring in general isn't good. It means you have an airway constriction while you are sleeping. Even the occasional snorer has an increased risk of high blood pressure, and the habitual snorer is much more likely to have high blood pressure.[3]

You can use the Cottle's maneuver to check your nasal airways. This is how you can tell where your airway blockage is causing labored inhalation:

1. Take two fingertips and place them on your cheek on one side of your nose.
2. Gently press down and pull away from your nose to open the air valve.
3. Take a breath in and see if you breathe easier.
4. Repeat this on the other side of your nose.

If you do breathe easier, you may need to try some nasal breathing strips at night (or even during the day) to help you breathe. This can often fix the problem, but you could have other issues requiring further steps from a doctor like a deviated septum or collapsed nasal valve.

One study showed that even the occasional snorer has around a 75 percent chance of having some form of sleep apnea.[4] There are some at-home testing units you can use to test for sleep apnea. They're not as good as a sleep study ordered by a physician, but they only cost about $100, and your insurance may cover it.

Oropharyngeal or myofunctional therapy exercises have been shown to help with snoring as well as reduce the severity of mild to moderate cases of obstructive sleep apnea syndrome (OSA).[5] Let's think of these exercises like training—you don't get ripped from going to the gym just one time, right? Doing these exercises consistently is likely to help you sleep better and breathe better. People who do these very simple exercises on a consistent basis for a few months can improve their OSA and snoring.[6] Most of these exercises are so easy and non-invasive you can do them while watching TV, scrolling social media, or, better yet, while you are working out that bod (double whammy!). The exercises will strengthen those floppy muscles we talked about earlier, which will reduce your snoring and OSA symptoms.[7]

Most research points to doing these exercises two to three times a day, and you can see and feel improvement within three months.[8] You may think that's such a long time before seeing results. But how long have you been breathing poorly? You can either try these minimum exercises for your breathing or get a massive CPAP machine to sleep with. The choice is yours.

So try to do a combination of the following exercises two to three times a day. Pick one a day and focus on that.

Tongue Exercises

1. Tongue slide: Place the tip of your tongue on the back of your upper front teeth. Slowly bring your tongue back, keeping the tip on the roof of your mouth, Repeat five to ten times.
2. Tongue stretch: Stick your tongue out as far as you can. Look at the ceiling and try to touch the tip of your chin with the tip of your tongue. Hold for ten to fifteen seconds and increase the duration as you can. Repeat five times.
3. Tongue push up: Press your entire tongue up against the roof of your mouth and hold it there for ten seconds. Repeat five times.
4. Tongue push down: Put the tip of your tongue against your lower front teeth and push the back of your tongue down against the floor of your mouth. Hold it there for ten seconds. Repeat five times.

Face Exercises

1. Cheek hook: Hook your right index finger inside your right cheek and gently pull outward. Then use your cheek muscles to try to pull your cheek back in. Repeat ten times on each side.
2. Pursed lips: Purse your lips to tightly close your mouth. Then open your mouth and relax your jaw and lips. Repeat ten times.

Repeating Vowel Sounds

Pronouncing vowel sounds uses the muscles in your throat, so repeating them can help strengthen those muscles.

Play around with saying each sound for *a*, *e*, *i*, *o*, and *u*, normally, stretching them out, and saying them slower or faster. Repeat each vowel ten to twenty times. You can also combine vowel sounds.

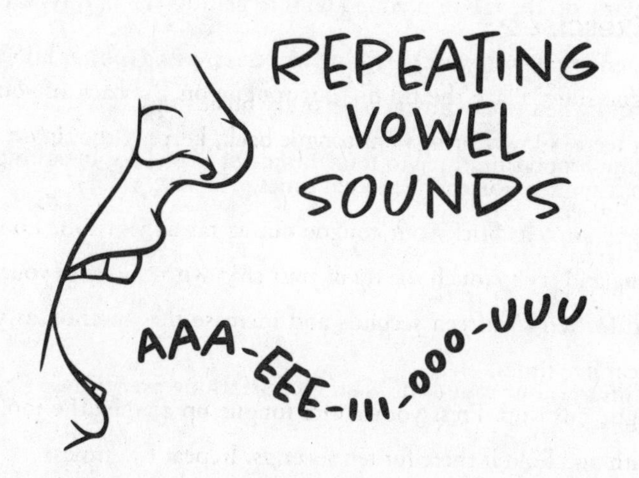

USING THE VOWEL SOUNDS A-E-I-O-U, PLAY AROUND WITH SAYING EACH NORMALLY, STRETCHING THEM OUT, SAYING THEM SLOWER OR FASTER, ETC. REPEAT THE SAME VOWEL 10-20 TIMES AND THEN CHANGE TO A DIFFERENT ONE. YOU CAN ALSO COMBINE VOWELS.

THE MINIMUM METHOD BREATHING PROTOCOLS

Let's Go!

- Work on breathing correctly—through your nose while expanding your stomach and then chest—for at least five to ten minutes every day.
- Use breathwork, whether it be physiological sighs or alternate nostril breathing, to alleviate stress.
- If you snore, start doing daily tongue and face exercises.

Level Up!

- Be mindful of your breathing throughout the day, and make sure you are breathing through your nose.
- Regularly do the CP test; your goal is to get to a CP of forty seconds.
- Be intentional with your breathing while exercising (power HISS breathing) and when you're finished (recovery breathing).
- Start incorporating three to four rounds of Wim Hof breathing at least once a week.

Max Out!

- Do three to four rounds of Wim Hof breathing every day.

5

EATING & NUTRITION

You Really Are What You Eat

Nutrition has become a ruthless element of the health industry. We have the vegans fighting with the carnivores, the keto believers saying they're better than paleo, and the calorie controllers thinking everyone else is crazy. How and why did we get to the point where we get so easily worked up over what other people eat?

In my opinion, we're focusing on the wrong thing. Most of what we are being told is what not to eat, and that can be really confusing. No, not all calories are created equal. The macronutrient (a.k.a. fats, proteins, and carbohydrates) and micronutrient (a.k.a. vitamins and minerals) ratio of an apple is very different from that of apple juice. But do most people really need to focus on all of that? I vote no.

I'm all about simplifying things. And no, I'm not about to feed you (pun intended!) all that moderation is key BS. The problem isn't that people are choosing not to moderate. The problem is that they can't moderate. Have you ever wondered why eating just one brownie turned into an all-night binge on sweets? It's because the sugar in the brownie creates a reptilian brain drug response similar to that of an addict who takes a hit of cocaine. Your brain gets flooded with dopamine, and it immediately wants more. This is why the concept of moderation doesn't work. You can't moderate a chemical addiction.

We need to fundamentally change the way we look at food and how we nourish our bodies. When it comes down to it, we are overcomplicating things. We are looking at the research all wrong and only reading the headlines. It's time to simplify nutrition. That's what we'll tackle in this chapter. As always, I want you to read the whole chapter so you can consume (pun intended!) all its nutritional goodness. But for all you short-on-time people, you can find the list of Minimum Method nutrition protocols at the end of the chapter.

For years, we've been told that salt causes high blood pressure. But when we look at the research, there is nothing that shows a direct cause of high blood pressure from excess amounts of sodium. Most of the studies that tie salt to high blood pressure looked at people who were taking all that salt from foods with high amounts of processed carbs, sugars, and fats. We're going to blame the salt and ignore all that other crap? That doesn't make sense. The same can be said for red meat and cholesterol. Is it crazy to assume that maybe the people eating a lot of red meat who have high cholesterol are also eating other foods that could be affecting their cholesterol?

The science community is famous for "knowing" things until it proves them otherwise. Remember the egg and cholesterol debate? How many years did we go back and forth on whether eggs are good or bad for cholesterol? Finally, the issue has been laid (again, pun intended!) to rest that eggs raise good HDL cholesterol and won't raise bad LDL cholesterol.

See what I mean. We aren't always looking at the full picture, and we aren't always looking without bias. Strip away all the science and go back to the early days of humankind. We have been living off animal products and plants for millions of years, and our bodies have learned to digest both. Our bodies do really well when we feed them real food. The problem is we've gotten too far away from eating real food. Our chemical addictions have us eating way too much processed food, which has made us overweight, unhealthy, and unhappy. So then what do we do to try to fix it? The infamous d-word.

How many times have you or someone you know said they were on a diet? I bet the word *diet* left a poor taste in your mouth, or you cringed a little when you heard it. That's because *diet* has a negative connotation in our society today. It insinuates that we are depriving ourselves of something we want. It often conjures feelings of being starved and miserable. And that's not an inaccurate reaction. The sad fact is that right now there are millions of people who are on a diet, yet they are completely unhealthy and continually gaining weight. That *is* miserable! But the truth is we are all on a diet.

The word *diet* merely refers to what you eat. So even if you eat like most Americans—a lot of soda, packaged food, and a lack of nutrients—you are on a diet whether you know it or not! You are on the standard American diet, or SAD. And that acronym couldn't be more fitting. First things first. We need to change the way we think of the word *diet*.

In this chapter, I'm not going to get into whether one diet is good or bad. Instead, I want you to simply focus on better ways to nourish and fuel your body and your mental state. These are general guidelines to help you reach better health. Ultimately, you have to find what works for you and what you'll realistically be able to stick to.

HOW YOU EAT MATTERS

Before we get into what you're eating, let's start with the act of eating itself. When was the last time you sat down to eat a meal and really took your time? Before you answer me, here is what I mean by taking your time. Whether you cooked your own meal or not (I'm assuming it's not), did you stop to look at your meal? Did you take a moment to truly enjoy how lucky you are to have this food that will (hopefully) nourish your body and brain? Did you turn off the TV? Did you take a moment to smell the aromas as you started salivating at the mere thought of enjoying your amazing meal? Be honest. I'm willing to bet the answer is no.

Here's what probably happens instead. You order out or zap a meal in Mr. Microwave, turn on the TV, and scarf down the food as fast as possible because you have things to do. Or you stopped by a drive-through or gas station and ate your meal as you were driving in traffic screaming at the a-hole who just cut you off while you were making a lane change with your knees. Did I nail it?

So what's my point? I'm going to let you in on a big secret that no one probably ever told you and was absent from the countless diet books and articles you've read. Digestion starts even before you take your first bite of food. Our bodies need to be ready to digest and absorb the nutrients from the meal we are about to eat, whether that is a candy bar or the healthiest organic meal on the planet. Of course I prefer it not to be a candy bar, but if you are going to eat it, you might as well digest the food and use it as energy as opposed to simply scarfing it down. Even if you are living off SAD, which is truly sad, I still want your food to be used to fuel your body, no matter how inefficient that fuel is. Let's change the meaning of SAD to *salivating and digesting.*

This beginning phase of digestion is called the cephalic phase. In Latin, *cephalic* means head, so think of eating with your head first. Your eyes, nose, ears, taste, and even thoughts start the digestion process. When you take a moment to look at your food, smell it, think about it, and even hear it being cooked, your body starts to release key digestive enzymes. The cephalic phase helps move you into a parasympathetic state. Eating while being in a sympathetic state, on the other hand, causes constriction of blood vessels, increased heart rate, constriction of intestinal and urinary sphincters, reduced intestinal activity, and reduced blood flow to the gut, muscles, and heart. This is exactly why you don't want to be stressed while eating—your body is fighting not to digest your food! Undigested food can do a number on your gut health, leading to bacterial overgrowth (not the good kind) and increased fermentation in the gut, causing stinky gas, indigestion, bloating, and constipation.

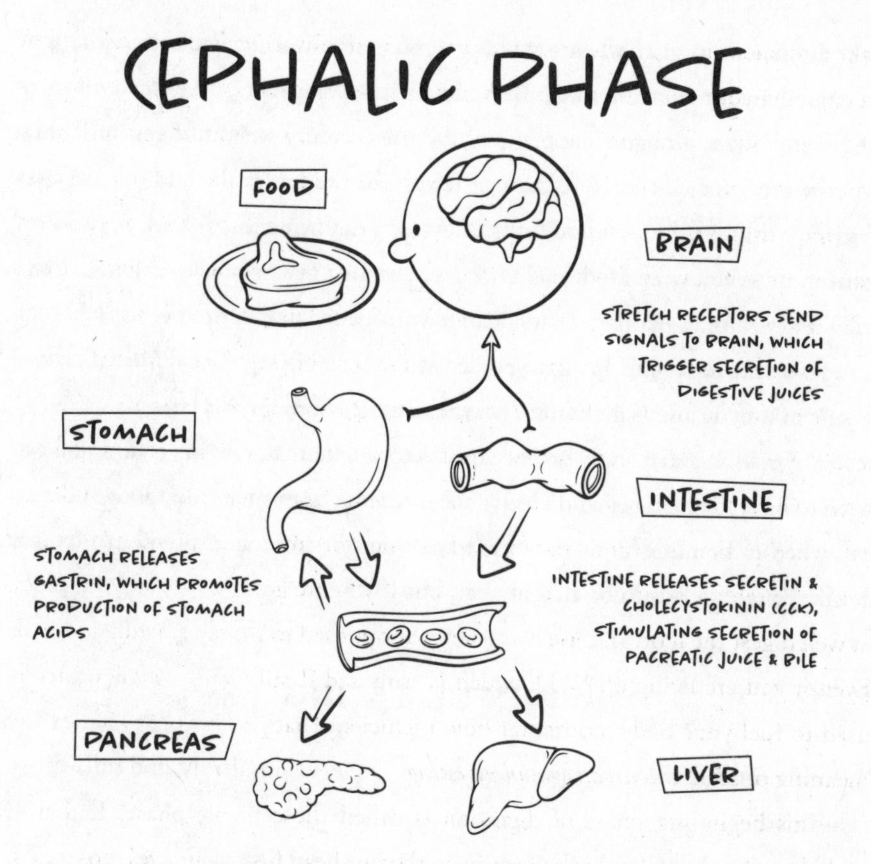

When we are stressed—and that includes being in a hurry—blood is redirected away from our stomachs to areas like our muscles because our body is in fight-or-flight mode. That inhibits digestion and messes with our gut microbiome. A review of twenty-three studies showed people who ate fast were almost twice as likely to be obese.[1] Why? It takes about twenty minutes for your brain to realize you are full. So when you scarf down your food, you're going to continue eating after you are technically full because of that lag time. If you eat while distracted, like while watching TV, it is likely you will consume anywhere from 10 percent to up to 50 percent more calories in an entire day.[2] Eating slowly and intentionally, on the other hand, changes your gut peptide response,[3] making it easier for you to know when you are satiated.

Studies show that when people pay more attention to what they eat, they consume 10 percent fewer calories.[4] You see, being attentive, as the authors of the study say, is a major piece in maintaining healthy weight, digestion, and a host of other factors. That 10 percent fewer calories can really add up. Let's say you typically eat the standard 2,000 calories a day while distracted. If you slow down and enjoy your food, and end up eating 10 percent fewer calories, that's 200 fewer calories per day. That adds up to 1,400 fewer calories per week, which can result in 20 pounds lost in a year! Now that's assuming the calorie deficit will result in weight loss, which isn't always the case. More on this later.

For now, the first thing you need to change about your eating is how you eat. Don't worry, we will get into food choices in a bit. But right now, above all else, you need to be mindful of your food and your environment so you can be in a relaxed state ready to fully digest your food.

MINDFUL EATING

Here are some tricks to help you slow down, eat more mindfully, and fully digest your food:

- Cook your own food (if possible): The mere act of prepping and cooking food will start to move you out of a sympathetic state and into a more relaxed state.
- Be present: Turn off all distractions like the TV and your phone, and take a minute or two to fully come into the moment of eating. Take a couple of deep breaths or do a breathing exercise from the breathing chapter if you need to.
- Be thankful: I know it might sound cheesy, but it works. Take a moment and be grateful for the food in front of you. Say it out loud. Remember, thinking about your food helps kick off your digestion process.
- Smell your food: Before you start eating, look at the food in front of you and smell it. I mean really smell it. Take a big breath in through

your nose—you should know the importance of that from the breathing chapter—and inhale the aromas of your meal.

- Take small bites: Don't shovel your food into your mouth. Use smaller silverware if you need to. Sometimes I use my son's fork or spoon to force me to take smaller bites.
- Chew slowly and fully: Stop swallowing chunks of food. I'm not going to tell you to count and chew a certain number of times. Just chew your food slowly and fully, until it resembles baby food. Chewing is actually really good for you. It releases serotonin, which makes you happier, and it releases epithelial growth factor, a polypeptide that stimulates the growth and repair of the epithelial tissue present in your saliva, which can heal and protect the gut lining and even help with symptoms of reflux.[5] The mere act of chewing your food more will allow your body to digest more nutrients like vitamins and minerals from the food.

If you're having a smoothie or yogurt or something that doesn't really involve chewing, eat a couple of nuts or something crunchy first to activate your digestion. You can also make it a point to "chew" your smoothie or yogurt and get the same effect.

- Pause between bites: Put your fork or spoon down after every bite. This helps you slow down.
- Enjoy your food no matter what it is: Whether it's pizza, sweets, or a salad, you need to be okay with whatever you are eating for your body to digest it properly. Feeling guilty while eating or fearing your food will derail your health efforts can have some of the worst impacts on your digestive system.

While reading this chapter, I want you to be aware of who you are and why you do what you do. Yes, I want you to do everything you can to be as healthy and happy as possible. But that doesn't mean you can't ever enjoy yourself or eat the occasional treat.

There is a condition known as orthorexia where people are so afraid of eating something they deem is bad for them that they have a lot of anxiety around what they eat at all times. That anxiety can lead to gut issues even if you're making the best food choices. This is one of the main reasons I hate the diet books that make you feel bad about yourself if you get off track. You are human and it is going to happen. And guess what? That's perfectly okay! The guilt you feel after eating those cookies is often worse for you than the cookies themselves. That being said, sometimes there are foods you should avoid forever or for a certain period of time if you have an allergy, autoimmune disorder, or need to heal your gut. And that brings us to a gut check.

Signs you may have orthorexia:

- You avoid going out to eat or even going to a friend's house for dinner.
- You worry about how clean or healthy food is.
- You spend a lot of time researching and thinking about food.
- You avoid a broad range of foods or ingredients that you deem unhealthy, such as carbs, gluten, sugar, nightshades, and legumes.
- You're afraid to eat even one meal that isn't on your meal plan.
- You feel the urge to give others nutritional advice or tell them what they should and shouldn't eat.
- You get preoccupied looking at your body in the mirror or measuring yourself.
- You refuse to consider anyone else's beliefs regarding nutrition.

YOUR METABOLISM AS YOU AGE

Let's also touch on metabolism and age real quickly, as I often hear people make comments (or excuses!) about how your metabolism slows as you age. Scientists looked at this exact issue, and it turns out it's not true.[6]

In our first year of life, we require about 50 percent more energy (relative to height and weight) than our parents do. After infancy, our energy needs start to drop by about 3 percent each year until we reach our twenties. It then remains pretty stable until our fifties. People tend to think that it's all downhill after thirty, but the truth is that weight gain in your thirties isn't because of a slowing metabolism. You can usually thank stress, lack of sleep, poor nourishment, and not enough physical activity for that. Our metabolism doesn't really slow down until after the age of sixty, when it starts to drop by about 0.7 percent each year. So by the time you're in your nineties, you need 26 percent fewer calories compared to your fifties. Now, part of that is usually due to a decrease in muscle mass, as people are less active and less likely to resistance train as they age. More reasons to use the tools in this book to keep your muscle mass as you age!

A QUICK GUT CHECK

Before we get into what to eat, I want you to take this quick gut health quiz. And be honest! Answer yes or no to the following questions:

- Do you pass foul-smelling gas more than ten times a day (especially after eating)?
- Do you often burp either before or after meals?
- Do you experience heartburn?
- Are you ever constipated or have loose stools, basically anything other than one long, soft piece (like a snake)?
- Do you have fewer than seven bowel movements per week (one per day)?
- Does it ever feel like you can't fully empty your bowels?
- Do you feel bloated after you eat?
- Do you need more than a few wipes with toilet paper to get clean?
- Do you often use antacids?
- Have you used antibiotics within the past six months?
- Do you constantly feel stressed?

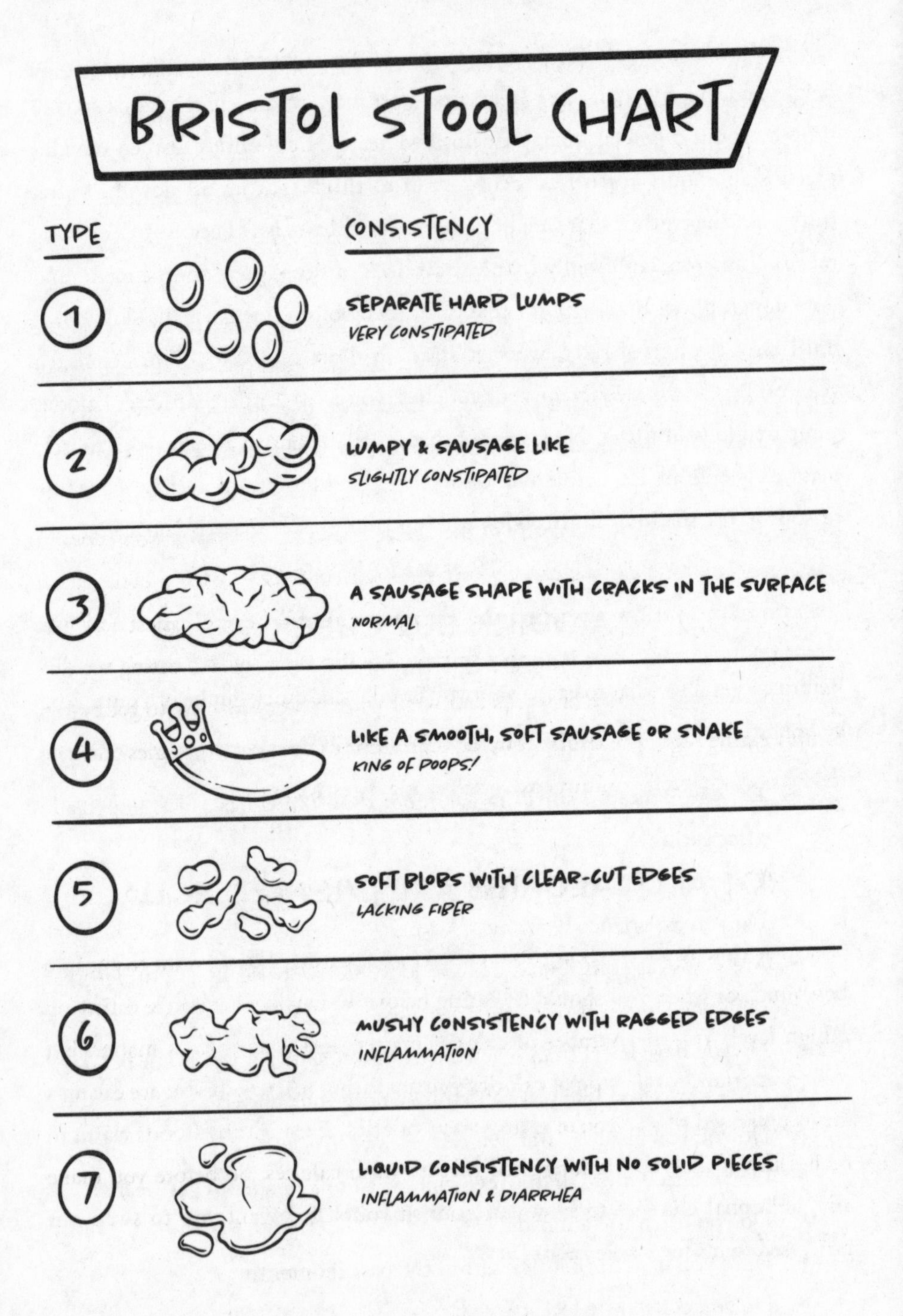
BRISTOL STOOL CHART
TYPE
CONSISTENCY
1
SEPARATE HARD LUMPS
VERY CONSTIPATED
2
LUMPY & SAUSAGE LIKE
SLIGHTLY CONSTIPATED
3
A SAUSAGE SHAPE WITH CRACKS IN THE SURFACE
NORMAL
4
LIKE A SMOOTH, SOFT SAUSAGE OR SNAKE
KING OF POOPS!
5
SOFT BLOBS WITH CLEAR-CUT EDGES
LACKING FIBER
6
MUSHY CONSISTENCY WITH RAGGED EDGES
INFLAMMATION
7
LIQUID CONSISTENCY WITH NO SOLID PIECES
INFLAMMATION & DIARRHEA

If you answered yes to more than two of the above, you may want to consider doing a gut reset to help with your gut health, microbiome, and gut lining.

You can also let your poop be your guide. Literally. Introducing the Bristol Stool Chart.[7] This chart was developed to help doctors gauge digestive health simply by looking at poop (or you telling them what it looks like).

Have you ever wondered what your poop should look like? The perfect consistency of poop is a long, soft snake (number 4 on the chart). If you have little hard pellets, it means you could be constipated, and your colon is not absorbing enough water. On the other end of the spectrum, if your poop is very soft or runny, it usually means you have symptoms of diarrhea, and too much water is being absorbed.

If you answered yes to many of the above questions, and your poop doesn't look like number 4 on the chart, don't freak out just yet. This is a book about the minimum you can do to get the maximum results. So the easiest and first change you should make is simply start practicing the mindful eating we discussed above for a couple of weeks and see if your symptoms start to get better. Simply eating more mindfully coupled with some of the sleep strategies outlined in the sleep chapter can immensely help your digestive system.

NOT ALL CALORIES ARE CREATED EQUAL

Okay, it's time to start talking about what you're eating. I don't want to get into how much or when you should be eating before we tackle what you're eating on a high level. Yes, the number of calories matter, and your macros matter, but more importantly, the type of calories you are eating matters. If you are eating a lot of processed foods, you're eating trash calories. Even if those foods claim to be healthy, if they have a long shelf life, it's trash calories. So before you make any additional changes to how you nourish yourself, I want you to swap out processed foods for whole foods.

First, let's be clear on what counts as processed food. Processed foods usually but not always come in a package. They are, as the name suggests, foods that go through a process, such as cookies, cakes, donuts, sodas, chips, frozen foods, and fried foods. These foods also have all sorts of ingredients in them to add color, make them shelf stable, add more taste, and ultimately make them addictive. They contain a lot of seed oils and emulsifiers to keep them from becoming solid (think salad dressing in your fridge). These emulsifiers promote inflammation and interfere with the body's ability to know if it is full or not, in turn making you eat more and more of these foods.

So why else are they so bad? Processed foods are thought to interrupt our gut microbiome and make our gut lining more permeable, which can lead to disorders like leaky gut, autoimmune diseases, a less diverse gut microbiome, and increased markers of inflammation, making it harder to fight off viruses and diseases.[8]

Processed foods also often lack fiber. Now, fiber isn't just what we need to take a poo; it is now thought to help feed our gut microbiome and mucosal lining. Fiber is an important food source for our good gut bacteria. Put it this way, if you aren't getting enough fiber, you are essentially starving your gut microbiome.

Still have doubts? Maybe you have lost weight eating junk food, but would you have done better with your weight loss (not to mention your bloodwork and markers) if what you had eaten were whole foods? The most recent study to date took a look at diet and food quality.[9] Two groups over twelve weeks had an energy restriction of 25 percent, which should lead to an overall weight loss really no matter what you eat. The people in one group had more freedom to eat what they wanted as long as they kept their calories to the 25 percent deficit. The high-nutrient group removed fructose (but not fruit!) and processed foods from their diet, consumed more fiber, omega-3 fats, plant protein, and monounsaturated fat. The results? Both groups lost weight but people following the high-quality diet lost 2.1 kilograms (4.62 pounds) more over the course of the twelve weeks!

Dan Garner is a functional medicine practitioner, nutrition coach, strength coach, and researcher who works with some of the top athletes in the world, including world champion UFC fighters. If he can get them into fight shape, the rest of us are easy peasy! This is what he has to say about fiber[10]:

> When it comes to applying something very simple and actionable to improve many different parameters of health, incorporating more fiber is absolutely one of the first things that comes to mind for me.
>
> Although fiber is technically within the world of carbohydrates, it serves very different functions than glucose and goes through a drastically different digestion and assimilation process, which results in a very different physiological outcome.
>
> There are two primary forms of dietary fiber: soluble and insoluble.
>
> Soluble fiber has the ability to dissolve in water. A good example here is guar gum. Add water to that and it will absorb the fluid and turn itself into a thick gel substance. Soluble fiber has a tendency to slow the movement of accompanying food through your GI tract and also is fermentable, which means it serves as a food source for your gut bacteria. Soluble fiber supplies your bacteria with their preferred energy source to maintain a healthy microbiome, while also adding bulk/substance to your stool in the process (i.e., if you have loose stools, soluble fiber is what is going to help turn them into healthy logs).
>
> The consumption of soluble fiber by the bacteria in the colon has also been shown to speed up fecal output as the bacteria themselves become healthier over time and become more proficient in the world of optimal digestion. Common sources of soluble fiber include beans, oats, apples, and sweet potatoes.
>
> Insoluble fiber, on the other hand, will not dissolve in water but will still contribute to stool weight/bulk. Insoluble fiber is the true "brush" going down your GI tract, sweeping the walls clean and getting rid of GI residue that doesn't belong there. Typical sources for insoluble fiber include the more "whole grain" style of foods

such as rice, amaranth, and bran. However, one of the best sources of insoluble fiber is avocado.

Now that we know what it is and where it comes from, why would we want to increase it in the first place?

Despite popular belief, fiber intake is tied to much more within our physiology than just helping us have regular bowel movements.

Although fiber isn't technically essential in any certain amount (meaning you don't need large amounts of it to live; Inuits are great examples of this), it doesn't mean it won't have positive benefits toward both your health and body composition. This is important to care about because many people will use the "fiber isn't essential" argument to somehow demonstrate that it doesn't have benefits, but this logic is flawed. Just because we can survive without it doesn't mean we can't thrive if we include it.

As I go through the myriad of benefits fiber offers the consumer, it's important to note that these benefits result through processes both in the upper and lower GI tract and are not as a result of just one particular section of the gut.

Research from the Institute of Social and Preventive Medicine in Switzerland found fiber intake to be associated with reduced risk of mouth and throat cancer.[11] Additional research at the Imperial College supported this evidence and found getting adequate fiber reduced overall breast cancer risk.[12]

As it relates to heart disease, researchers found that each 10 grams increase in fiber intake was associated with a 14 percent decrease in the risk of all heart disease and a 27 percent decrease in the risk of death resulting from heart disease.[13]

With respect to metabolic syndrome, blood sugar regulation, and type 2 diabetes, increasing your daily fiber intake is one of the most powerful things you can do. There is plenty of excellent data demonstrating fiber's ability to significantly reduce cholesterol, improve blood sugar control, and reduce blood pressure.

Fiber also creates one of the most effective satiety signals within the body, giving you the feeling of fullness and satisfaction both in the short and long term. This is important to care about as we can then manipulate fiber content of certain foods to either promote satiety or reduce it.

In a couple examples, we would promote satiety in those looking to lose weight, preferably in the evening when cravings tend to be the greatest. On the other side of the fence, it would be wiser to lower daily fiber intake for those looking to gain weight and find it tough to get all the calories in.

More fiber means less appetite, and less fiber means more appetite. So whether you want to gain weight or lose it, fiber can help you from a consistency perspective since it impacts the quality of your state of mind with respect to hunger signals.

Fiber's satiety is created through two different mechanisms:

1. Physically stretching the gut walls and activating stretch receptors, which send chemical signals to the brain telling you that you're full.
2. Slowing gastric emptying.

Number 1 is quite obvious in its mechanism, but number 2 is a big reason why fiber has done so well in the blood glucose control research. Slowing the rush of sugar into the bloodstream allows for a much more manageable and smooth absorption process, diffusing any of the large spikes and crashes that you would normally see in the absence of fiber.

Last but not least, in case you needed another reason to get on the fiber train, excellent research has demonstrated that probiotic supplementation benefits are limited by the amount of fiber you consume in your whole food diet.[14] Meaning, if you don't consume enough fiber, your probiotic supplement is genuinely useless within your body.

So, how do we get some in our diet, and how much of it should we aim for on a daily basis? Our target is to consume 10 grams of fiber per 1,000 calories per day, and you can go the supplement route or the food route.

Utilizing supplementation is a very easy and cost-effective strategy, psyllium husk being your main go-to weapon of choice.

However, I'm always a fan of prioritizing whole foods so incorporating a balanced intake between the above options of soluble and insoluble fiber intake before relying on supplementation is preferred due to the many other benefits that whole foods provide.

If you're currently nowhere near 10 grams of fiber per 1,000 calories per day, you don't want to go up to this amount overnight as it will create a lot of gastrointestinal distress. I have found through coaching thousands of clients that adding an additional 5 grams per week into your diet until you reach this target allows you to receive all of the benefits with none of the initial negative side effects.

Additionally, research suggests it typically takes up to four weeks for fiber to alter your microbiome in a positive way, anyway, so the "slow and steady" process makes sense from all angles as you gain nothing from going too hard too soon.

Patience is key. Enjoy!

So, case in point, you should stay away from processed foods. But I don't want you to think you can never have french fries, chips, or a donut again in your life. Let's be real here! I would prefer you make them yourself, but that's probably not realistic, either. You are going to have them on occasion, and that is okay! The goal is to make the vast majority of your diet whole foods instead of processed foods.

Take it from Dr. James DiNicolantonio, author of *The Salt Fix*. He says[15]:

> One of the simplest things people can do to lose weight is to go through their kitchen cabinet and throw out the junk food. Half the battle with weight loss is eliminating the bad food and the other half is eating healthy whole foods. For example, one study took twenty adults and instructed them to consume as much or as little food as desired either from ultra-processed foods or unprocessed foods for two weeks immediately followed by the alternate diet.[16] Subjects who consumed the ultra-processed foods ended up eating 508 calories more per day

compared to those eating unprocessed foods. Additionally, those eating the ultra-processed foods gained two pounds of body weight, whereas those eating the unprocessed foods lost two pounds. This highlights the fact that the quality of the food you eat determines how many calories you eat and how much weight you gain.

You see, I really don't care about how many calories you are eating if they are coming from processed foods. Make an effort and simply start eating foods that don't have an ingredient list. Think blueberries—you know what their ingredient is? Blueberries! Wild-caught salmon, greens, potatoes—you get the point. No need to get into the weeds yet. Just start eating more whole foods and less trash.

Now, once you have done that, if your digestive symptoms still persist, it may be a good idea to try an elimination diet to give your gut a reset. Many foods can trigger symptoms of poor health, but the opposite is also true—adding more good foods into your diet can often help with your digestive health. This is something I don't think is talked about enough.

RESET YOUR GUT: THE BELLY BOUNCE BACK

If you have no digestive issues whatsoever and are calm while you slowly eat your food, then you can probably skip this section. However, a gut cleanse to reset your gut can still help identify any food sensitivities you may not be aware of. As long as you are honest with yourself and how you feel after you eat a food, you can often pinpoint which foods bother you. Now, this can be easier said than done because we rarely eat one food at a time. But you can usually notice patterns when you feel like crap after you eat a certain type of food. For me, it's artificial sweeteners and sugar alcohols. That's why even certain types of protein powder (which are seemingly healthy) will wreck my stomach so much that I'm clearing out the room with my gas and waking myself up farting . . . yeah, that's a thing. So I know to always check ingredients for artificial sweeteners and sugar alcohols.

So here is an elimination diet protocol to help you understand your body more. In an elimination diet, you omit major allergen foods from your meals and slowly reintroduce them after thirty days. So you may not have to say goodbye to one of your favorite foods forever; just goodbye for now to see what the issue is and help heal your gut. Resetting your gut is a great way to get more in tune with your body as well as eat a lot of whole foods while getting creative with adding them into your diet. This is not a weight loss diet, but it is likely you will lose weight by taking away major food allergens and decreasing inflammation. I'm not going to give you a calorie range here, simply nourish and fuel with real food! Do your best to stay the course, and if you go off track for one meal or bite, just own it and move on!

Here's the thing. I prefer you stick to this 100 percent, but we all mess up every now and then. For example, it's likely that in the first few days you eat something that you forgot had nuts in it or had a sauce with honey. That's okay. I don't need you to go back to day one; just keep on moving. If you accidentally eat gluten on day twenty and feel like death, then you know that gluten probably caused a reaction. Get back to the plan and take a note of that body response. But if you find yourself constantly struggling to stay on this program and eating what you're not supposed to, then maybe it's not for you. And that's okay, too.

You may want to ease into this and simply start taking out processed foods, alcohol, and sugars, but if you are a hit-the-ground-running type of person, then have at it! It's important that you stop taking any NSAIDs, if possible, while resetting your gut, and do not do this if you are taking antibiotics, as they will do a number on your gut all by themselves.

The Thirty-Day Belly Bounce Back

Day 1–30

Eliminate the following foods:

- Carbs: Gluten and legumes, including beans.
- Processed meats: Hot dogs and bacon.

- High-mercury fish: Tuna, swordfish, and lobster.
- Soy and soybeans.
- Sweeteners: Natural sweeteners, such as sugar, honey, agave, corn syrup, and brown sugar; and artificial sweeteners, such as aspartame, sorbitol, neotame, and saccharine. Basically, if it adds sweetness and isn't fruit, don't have it.
- Additives: MSG and dyes. In fact, it's a good idea to never eat these.
- Seed oils (the hateful eight): Corn, cottonseed, canola, grape, sunflower, sesame, soybean, and safflower.
- Non-water beverages: Sodas (including diet sodas), juices, energy drinks, alcohol, milk, and caffeine. If you absolutely need your caffeine, you can have a little coffee or organic tea, but try to taper off each week. For example, if you usually have three cups of coffee per day, do that for the first week then try to cut back to two cups in week two, one cup in week three, and zero cups for the remainder of the time. Or you can get down to half a cup when you really need it, like before you train or when you need a quick shot in the ass for productivity.
- Eggs: Yes, eggs are good for you but can cause a reaction in many people.
- Nuts: Nuts also have a place in a healthy eating plan but often cause issues (bloating, constipation, the runs, and other GI distresses) with some people. Removing nuts from your diet for a certain period of time can help.
- Dairy: People often have an issue with dairy because of its lactose.
- Prebiotic supplements & food: These are good for you, but prebiotics can cause issues for people with IBS and make symptoms worse. If you have small intestinal bacterial overgrowth (SIBO) or fermentable oligosaccharides, disaccharides, monosaccharides, and polyols intolerance, then stay away as well. Examples of prebiotic foods include leeks, asparagus, artichokes, onions, garlic, corn, bananas, oats, and chicory root.

- Raw veggies . . . kind of: I hate even writing this because I believe vegetables have a great place in our eating plan. But if you have GI issues, raw vegetables can be harder to digest than cooked veggies. Now, do not read this and think that I said you shouldn't eat vegetables. On the contrary, just be aware that steaming vegetables, adding them to a pressure cooker or oven might help your gut a little. If you feel great after eating raw veggies, then go on with your bad self!
- Spicy food, chocolate, and red sauces like marinara: If you have acid reflux, remove these foods from your diet.

All right, I know you're all probably wondering what can you eat. Fair question. Here's what I want you eating for the first thirty days of the gut cleanse:

- Cooked veggies: You can have raw vegetables if you know you can handle them well. Some people may handle leafy greens better than something denser like broccoli, beets, carrots, green peas, and parsnips.
- Meat: Preferably organic and grass fed. No processed meats.
- Fruit.
- Gluten-free grains: Quinoa, quinoa pasta, white rice, brown rice, wild rice, oats.
- Tubers: Potatoes and yams.
- Fats: Avocados, olives, extra-virgin olive oil (not for cooking), and avocado oil (can be used for cooking).
- Any food product that has all good ingredients and none of the ones on the remove list. A lot of food companies have gotten really good about making diet-friendly products for specific diets.

Okay, so you might be feeling super overwhelmed right now. I get it! But remember, this book is ultimately about doing what is best for you and not shaming you into anything. If all of the above feels impossible, just do what you can. Or, again, just focus on removing processed foods and eating more whole foods. The main goal is to start reading the labels on everything and being better informed about what's in the food you're eating. Ultimately, I would love for you to get to the point where none of the food you're eating even has a label!

I want to point out that a lot of elimination diets give you calorie restrictions as well. I'm not going to do that. Instead, I want you to focus on removing the foods listed above and eating as much as you want of the allowable foods. And if you can, try to diversify your foods as much as possible instead of eating the same foods every day. Variety is great for nutrient diversity and microbiome health.

Again, the goal of this diet isn't to lose weight, but you likely will shed a few pounds due to the increase in fiber and nutrients and decrease in inflammation. If you'd rather maintain or gain weight, then be sure to load up on approved carbs, healthy fats, and proteins. The bottom line is make this your own and remember you are eliminating foods in order to gain better health.

It is a sad fact that it is cheaper to eat unhealthy food. Processed foods often cost much less than whole foods, and your bank account may feel that when you start making the switch. Think of this as an investment in you and your health. You may be spending more on the front end, but you'll be saving a lot on the back end in both dollars and quality of life. Heart disease, diabetes, obesity, and other health issues end up costing a lot in doctors' visits, medications, and more.

After Day 30—Begin Reintroducing Foods

After thirty days, start reintroducing one food that you removed every three days. Eat a few servings of that food just on the first of the three days—don't have any more of that food on day two and three. Record how you feel each day. If you don't experience any symptoms, you can keep that food in your eating plan. If you have any kind of reaction, then don't eat that food again. Introduce foods in the following order:

Day 31–33: Eggs. Remember, have two to three servings of eggs on day thirty-one and no eggs on day thirty-two and thirty-three. Record your symptoms.

Day 34–36: Gluten and wheat. You can skip this category if you want to. Remember, there are a lot of options for breads and pastas that don't have gluten like potato bread and cassava.

Day 37–39: Beans and other legumes. You may have heard about antinutrients in certain foods like beans and legumes. Antinutrients are compounds in foods that can limit your body's ability to absorb certain nutrients. I don't want this book to be confusing so here's the bottom line: yes, antinutrients are a real thing, but they aren't a concern for most people because they are typically cooked out of the food.

Day 40–42: Nuts. Back to the antinutrient thing. Sorry, I have to cover my bases. The antinutrients found in nuts are oxalates and phytates. But simply soaking them in water and salt or lemon juice overnight then rinsing them in the morning can take care of a lot of the antinutrients. Honestly, my favorite is soaked almonds with some sea salt on them. They are a little chewy and delicious! You can even toss them in the oven afterward for a good crunch if you want. Many companies now sell presoaked and dried nuts.

Day 43–45: Raw veggies. If you didn't remove raw veggies, then skip this and move on to the next category.

Day 47–49: Caffeine and coffee. If you cut or decreased your caffeine intake, the same rules apply for reintroducing caffeine—slowly increase the amount you drink. So I would start with just one cup on day 47. If you don't have a reaction, you can slowly increase your caffeine intake over the next couple of weeks.

Day 50–52: Dairy. Ah, the dairy conundrum. You can opt to keep dairy out of your diet as long as you are getting enough calcium, vitamin D, and other nutrients found in dairy from other sources. Again, most people who have an issue with dairy have a problem with the lactose in the dairy. In fact, about 75 percent of the world's population is lactose intolerant. There is a lot of research on whether we need dairy, and while I don't think we need it, that doesn't mean you can't have it. Here's my advice: if you are going to consume dairy, make sure it is organic, hormone-free, and from a reputable source.

It's important to understand that not all dairy is created equal. For example, milk has much more lactose than butter, which has almost none. So if you are concerned about lactose but you still want to have dairy, here are your dairy go-tos:

- Butter and clarified butter (ghee) have extremely low levels of lactose or no lactose.
- Aged cheese such as cheddar, Swiss, and parmesan because the aging process further breaks down the lactose.
- Probiotic yogurt has live bacteria in it, which is able to break down lactose much easier. Studies show that people who have issues with milk are much less likely to have issues with yogurt.[17] Look for a yogurt that has "probiotic" on its label, which means it contains live cultures. The pasteurized versions do not have live cultures. Greek yogurt (shout-out to my in-laws and 50 percent of my son) has lower lactose, as the straining removes the whey and in turn brings down the lactose content.
- Dairy protein powder often has little to no lactose. Look for the isolate that has the lowest level of lactose.

Track your symptoms after eating dairy just as you did with the other foods, but also be aware when you add a source with a higher lactose content and record how you feel. If you cut out dairy altogether, you can replace it with foods that have a high amount of calcium and other nutrients typically found in dairy, such as sardines, figs, bok choy, kale, seaweed, almonds, oranges, sesame seeds, oatmeal, and collard greens.

Once you complete all of the above, you should have a good sense of what foods cause poor reactions. From there, it's up to you how often you eat those foods. If you think the food is worth the stomach issues, then at least you are making an informed and intentional decision. Just be smart about it.

OKAY, TIME TO COUNT CALORIES

Every person has a basal metabolic rate (BMR) that is essentially the number of calories a body burns in a day simply to maintain normal bodily functions. It's not referring to calories needed for normal daily activities like moving, walking, exercising, or even fidgeting. Yes, fidgeting burns calories!. It's only referring to the energy your body needs to stay alive. Basically, it's the calories you would burn if you just lay on your couch all day binging Netflix.

So your BMR is your baseline when it comes to calorie counting and your calorie burn. You are always going to burn that number of calories in a day. When you move more, you burn more calories (obviously). Even what are called thermogenesis activities like fidgeting, taping your feet, or nervous movement habits count toward your calorie burn. When you add more muscle, you increase your calorie burn because muscle requires more calories.

Ultimately, weight loss or gain does come down to the whole calories in vs. calories out thing, but in my opinion that matters less if you are eating the SAD diet. Again, I don't want you to worry about or count a single calorie until you put down the processed food and start eating whole foods that don't have an ingredient list or a marketing department pushing them. It is true that you can lose weight eating less of that shit, but it won't be quality weight. You will lose muscle, and you will be nutrient deficient eating that terrible diet even if it is fewer calories in than calories out.

So how do you determine how many calories you should be consuming in a day? Well, before we determine calories in, we need to determine calories out, a.k.a. your metabolic rate. Your metabolic rate is the number of calories (or the amount of energy) you burn on a daily basis. There are several ways to figure out your metabolic rate, and some are easier than others. If you want to get super legit and scientific, you can google *resting metabolic rate* or *resting energy expenditure (REE) testing near me* and go to breathe in and out of a tube to get your exact metabolic rate. These tests are the gold standard in metabolism testing and are usually inexpensive.

But the majority of people aren't going to do that, and I get it. Luckily, there are several different equations you can use to determine your BMR and how many calories you should consume daily based on your activity level. Here's a really simple one called the Mifflin-St. Jeor equation:

Men: (4.536 × weight in pounds) + (15.88 × height in inches) - (5 × age in years) + 5

Women: (4.536 × weight in pounds) + (15.88 × height in inches) - (5 × age in years) - 161

Find your BMR and then multiply by below.

BMR × 1.2: If you are sedentary, doing little to no exercise in a day

BMR × 1.375: If you are slightly active, doing light exercise or sports one to three days a week

BMR × 1.55: If you are moderately active, doing moderate exercise or sports three to five days a week

BMR × 1.725: If you are very active, doing hard exercise or sports six to seven days a week

BMR × 1.9: If you are extra active, doing very hard exercise or sports and a physical job or 2× training

So, a moderately active thirty-five-year-old cis woman weighing 150 pounds at 5'5", would have a BMR of 1,376 × 1.55, which would come to 2,132 calories daily to maintain her weight.

If math isn't your thing, you can simply google *total daily energy expenditure* or *TDEE calculator* and just plug in your information.

Now, I know that many of you are probably wondering if you really need to count calories. I say yes and no. Not a clear answer, I know, but here's what I mean. I recommend (again) that you count your calories for a couple of weeks to give you a good idea of what your daily count is. Then you'll be fine eyeballing your food intake.

The number of calories isn't the only factor that matters when discussing calories in. This is where your macros come into play and is another area where there is a lot of debate, but here's my stance on it. If you hit your protein requirements (which we will discuss below), then I don't really care if the rest of your calories

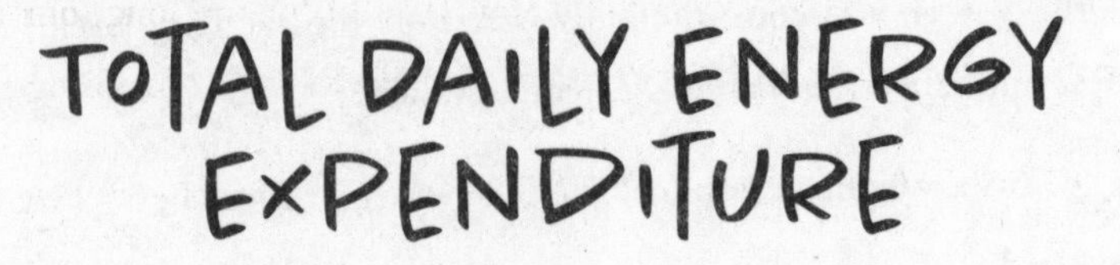

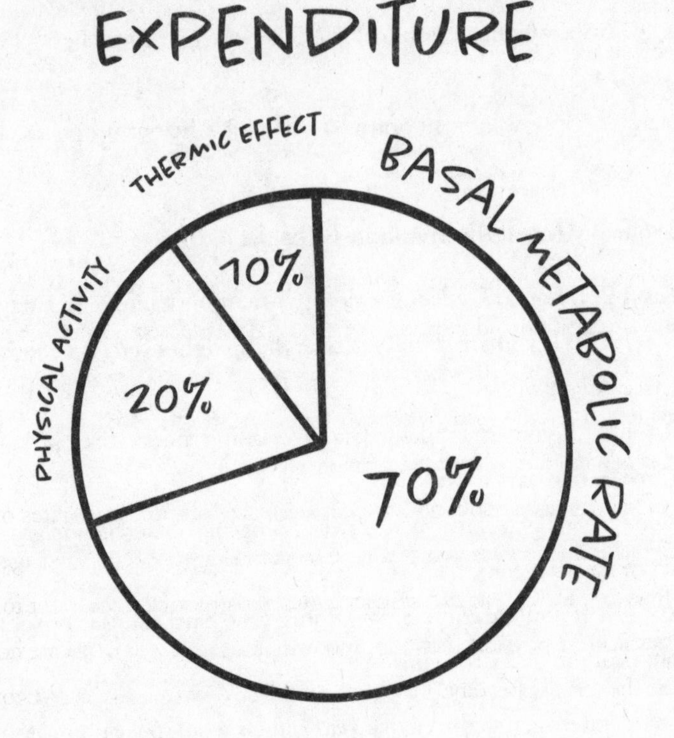

come from fat or carbs. You read that right—carbs are okay! Now, if you're a professional athlete, and your career depends on your performance, then we need to dial things in more. But for the everyday person wanting to be healthy, as long as your protein remains constant, you can vary your carbs and fat. Then, stay consistent and monitor the scale.

If you want to lose weight, cut your calories from carbs and fat (not protein!) for a couple of weeks and see how the scale responds. You only need to cut it by a little bit. I recommend only decreasing by 10 percent at a time, and each time monitor the scale for a couple of weeks before making any more adjustments. I recognize that 10 percent doesn't seem like a lot and that most diet plans and books call for much more drastic decreases. And to that I pose the following question to you and society as a whole—how's that working? Have we all gotten healthier and more fit? Not at all.

When we drastically cut calories too quickly and for too long, our bodies adapt metabolically to rely on less energy, fewer calories, and risk losing muscle tissue as well. That means you'll burn fewer calories and any excess is more likely to be stored as fat. This is why people say they wrecked their metabolism. It can take some effort to get back to that higher metabolic rate. Making small adjustments at a time is critical to maintaining your metabolic rate and ensuring you lose weight in a healthy way.

When you're trying to lose weight, you want to lose fat, not muscle. Cutting 10 percent of your calories is not only sustainable, but it's also usually super simple, like cutting out one tablespoon of olive oil. Then if you add more movement to your days—go for a walk after a meal, stand up during the day more often, or simply just fidget more—you can easily reach the magic goal of a 3,500-calorie deficit per week so many diet books promote.

One of my favorite resources for people is the National Institutes of Health Body Weight Planner, where you can type in your height, weight, and age, and get your BMR with TDEE. You can also set a goal weight, when you want to reach it, and what additional physical activities you will do, and it will calculate how many calories you should eat per day. To check it out, go to www.niddk.nih.gov/bwp.

A note on Body Mass Index (BMI). I, like many health experts, don't believe in the BMI scale because it doesn't take muscle tissue into account. It simply looks at height and weight. Even though I typically have a body fat percentage in the single digits, according to my BMI, I am considered overweight. The BMI scale was developed so insurance companies would have an easy way to assess their customers' risks. It holds no real value in indicating your health or fitness level. So my advice to you is to completely ignore it and always use body fat percentage instead.

I want your biggest takeaway from this section to be that small changes can yield big results, especially when it comes to your diet. You can't exercise away a bad diet so before you start hitting the gym more, we need to tighten up your diet.

Which foods your calories come from is a complicated topic. While different people will do better on different eating plans, I do believe there are some similarities in what most people should eat. If you did the elimination diet above, then you should know what specific foods you shouldn't eat. But I recommend everyone limit the following as much as possible:

- Alcohol.
- Sugar.
- Seed oils.
- Sugar alcohols like erythritol, glycerol, and isomalt that are often found in sugar-free and no-sugar-added foods that are still somehow sweet.

Those are my big no-no's. As for what you should be eating, I'm only going to take a hard stance on one thing—protein. Whether you're counting calories or not, I want you to pay attention to how much protein you eat. Okay, let's address the elephant in the room, as I'm sure many of you have seen a vegan post somewhere saying that you can easily get your daily protein needs from broccoli. Let me be clear—I'm not knocking vegans, and I'm not knocking broccoli. I'm a fan of both. But that protein strategy isn't optimal because broccoli—and all its cruciferous counterparts—is not a complete source of protein.

Let's dig into protein more.

PRIORITIZING PROTEIN

Why do I want you to focus on protein? Because protein has been shown to help with muscle tissue growth, healthy aging, satiety, weight management, and performance, among other things. It actually helps with athletic performance in and out of the gym by helping your muscles rebuild after you train. Plus, how many times have you heard someone of a certain age group fall and break a hip or something? That happens because of a loss of muscle tissue (a.k.a. sarcopenia) and bone density due to insufficient protein. So the bottom line is your body needs protein.

The current recommended dietary allowance (RDA) of protein is 0.8 grams of protein per kilogram of bodyweight. That usually equates to about 50 to 75 grams of protein per day, and it's just not enough. Then why is it the RDA? Without getting into the weeds, the recommendation was set based on nitrogen balance—which is not a good measure of protein needs—and is really only sufficient if you're a total couch potato . . . which I hope I've convinced you not to be by this point. The 0.8 grams of protein per kilogram of body weight is essentially the amount of protein you need to stay alive if you're just lying around all day. In my opinion, the RDA for protein is total crap (yes, I said it, come at me!).

Before I get into my protein recommendations, let me put any concerns to rest. There is no evidence that consuming more protein than the RDA will result in any issues[18] like renal disease[19] or adverse bone health.[20] So if you've heard that eating more protein than is recommended is bad for you in some way, know that is simply not true. In fact, if you already have some kind of kidney issue or decline in renal function, eating more protein and working out has actually shown to limit some of the negative symptoms.[21] Important note: if you have any health issues, always consult with your physician before changing your diet or lifestyle.

People used to think that excess calories of any macronutrient would lead to fat gain, but that is not true of protein. The extra amino acids from protein will cause weight gain, but not as much fat gain. A 2012 study overfed three different groups of people by 1,000 calories per day.[22] There was a high-protein group (25 percent of total calories), mid-protein group (15 percent of total calories), and low-protein group (5 percent of total calories). At the end of the study each group had gained a similar amount of weight, but the high-protein group gained less fat and more lean tissue.

A general protein target should be 1.2 to 1.6 grams of high-quality protein per kilogram (or 2.2 pounds) of body weight per day. This range has been shown to optimize your health better than the current crappy RDA.[23] So someone who weighs 150 pounds would eat from 81.8 grams (327 calories) to 109 grams (436 calories) of high-quality protein per day.

Here are protein requirements based on some goals:

- Athlete: 1.4 to 2.0 grams[24] per kilogram (or 2.2 pounds) of body weight.
- Bodybuilder/heavy-weight lifter: 1.7 to 2.2 grams[25] per kilogram (or 2.2 pounds) of bodyweight. The largest meta-analysis on protein and athletes shows the best protein range for muscle mass, strength, and to maximize lean mass is 1.6 to 2.2 grams[26] per kilogram (or 2.2 pounds) of body weight.
- Muscle gain: 1.6 to 2.4 grams[27] per kilogram (or 2.2 pounds) of body weight. For muscle gain with less fat gain[28] (for experienced lifters), studies suggest that assuming a hypercaloric state of 370 to 800 calories above maintenance will result in less fat gain due to the ratio of protein to other macros.
- Fat loss: 1.6 to 2.4 grams[29] per kilogram (or 2.2 pounds) of body weight. When resistance training in a caloric deficit, protein intake of 2.3 to 3.1 grams[30] per kilogram (or 2.2 pounds) of body weight resulted in more calories burned.

Please note that the above says *fat loss*. We don't simply want to lose weight. That is the wrong way of thinking. We want to lose fat and maintain muscle tissue. Muscle is more metabolically active, helps with insulin control, increases mobilization of fat, increases the use of fat for energy, helps us move better, decreases risk of injuries, makes our bones stronger, helps our mental health, increases our balance, and pretty much makes us superheroes.

On average, the leaner you are and more muscle tissue you have, the more protein you need to maintain that muscle tissue. That's not a hard-and-fast rule but something to keep in mind. In general, consuming around a gram of protein per pound of body weight is a good starting point. You can then play around with the numbers based on your goals and activity levels. But it's important to increase your protein amount gradually. Don't go from little protein to an extreme amount in one day. Instead, add a little more protein each day so that your body and digestive system can adapt to the change.

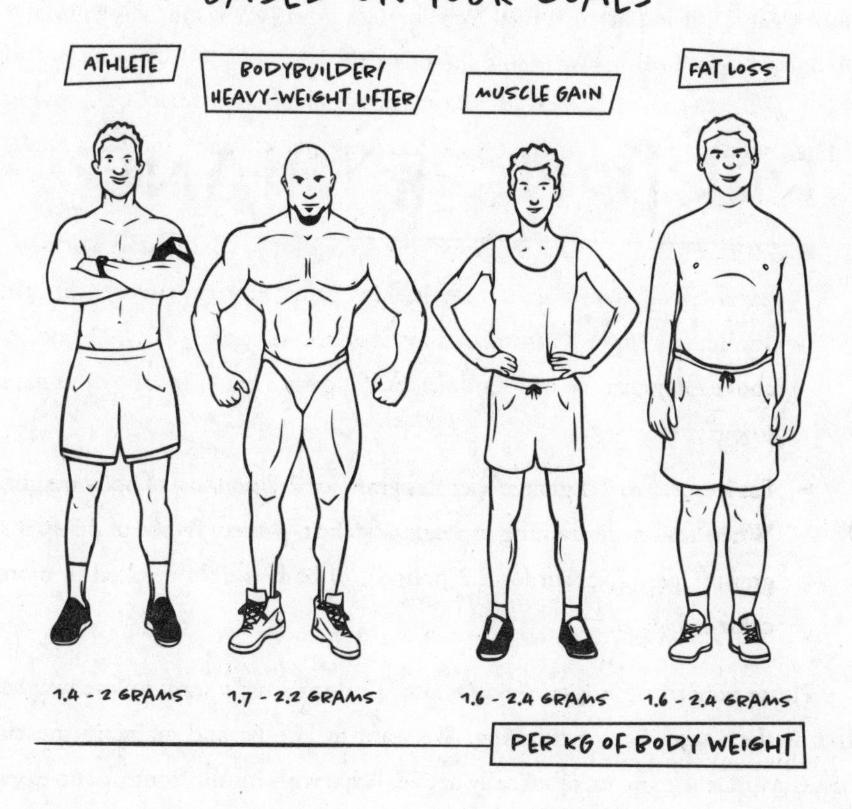

Once you find your ideal protein amount, you can fill in the rest of your calories with fats, carbs, or a combination of both. Yes, you read that correctly—you can have carbs. But not just any crappy carb or fat. I want you to nourish and fuel with healthy carbs and fats.

ON YOUR PLATE

Food scales and measuring cups aren't for everyone. But you do need some method of monitoring your portions. I like to keep it simple and use the most readily available measuring technique there is—my hands! At a minimum, your plate should look like this: a thumb-size portion of healthy fat, two palm-size portions of protein, a palm-size portion of healthy carbs, and a palm-size portion of fruits. If you stick with that as your minimum, you are on your way to maximum results! Oh and here is a treat for you, if it's green, eat as much as you want! No one ever got fat from asparagus and broccoli!

PORTIONS BY HAND

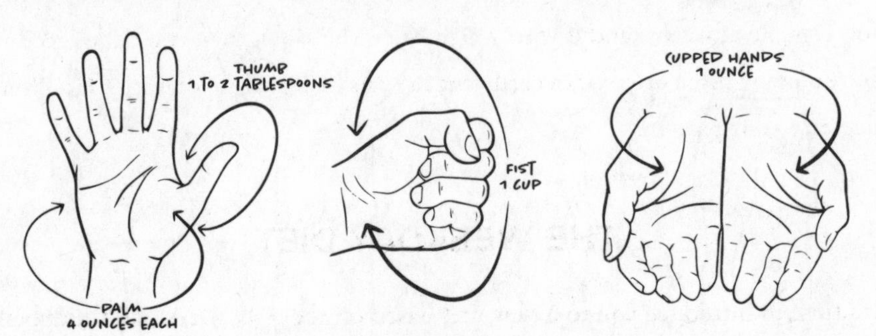

ONE MEAL

PROTEIN: 2 PALMS | VEGETABLES: 1 FIST | DENSE CARBS: 1 CUPPED HANDFUL
FRUIT: 1 CUPPED HANDFUL | FAT: 2 THUMBS

This could be a meal option for you:

- 2 palm-size portions of protein (chicken breasts): 187 calories, 35 g protein, 4 g fat
- 1 cupped handful of fruit (berries): 84 calories, 1 g protein, 4 g fiber, 21 g carbs
- 1 fistful of vegetables (spinach): 41 calories, 6 g protein, 5 g fiber, 7 g carbs
- 2 thumbs of fat (almonds): 102 calories, 4 g protein, 2 g fiber, 4 g carbs, 9 g fat
- 1 cupped handful of carbs (cooked quinoa): 222 calories, 8 g protein, 5 g fiber, 40 g carbs, 3 g fat
- Totals for one meal: 636 calories, 54 g protein, 72 g carbs, 16 g fiber, 16 g fat

Eating this three times a day will give you: 1,908 calories, 162 grams of protein, 48 grams of fiber, 223 grams of carbs, and 48 grams of fat. This keeps you at around 2,000 calories per day and meets the protein needs of most individuals. But as we discussed in the previous chapter, depending on how active you are, your body composition, and your BMR, you may need more or less calories than the example above.

Remember that protein needs to be your priority. Start by increasing or decreasing your protein accordingly. Then I recommend keeping the fruits and vegetables the same and bumping the carbs up or down as needed. Stick to this for a couple of weeks, and if your weight stays the same, then you either need to start moving more or you can easily cut calories by eating less carbs or fat. Don't decrease your protein.

THE WEEKDAY DIET

It's time to introduce you to a new diet based on the research of Bill Campbell, PhD, who studies the best methods for losing fat and gaining muscle. I call it The Weekday Diet. If you are like most people, you can eat pretty well during the week and then on the weekends you seem to go off the rails. That's why it's time we had a diet that allowed for some weekend fun!

Dr. Campbell ran a study for seven weeks with resistance-trained men and women (yes, resistance training is key to this diet working). The constants during the study were that all participants ate about one gram of protein per pound of body weight each day, and all participants resistance trained an average of twenty-four days out of the seven weeks (about three to four days a week). The variables during the study were one group of participants ate at a constant 25 percent calorie deficit for the whole seven weeks. The other group ate at a 35 percent deficit for five days during the week and then back up to the maintenance calories for the remaining two days, which averaged out to a 25 percent caloric deficit over the seven days. During those two days, they increased their carbohydrate intake.

What did Dr. Campbell and his colleagues find? Both groups lost weight, but there were some key differences.[31] The people in the group who increased their calorie and carb intake for two days better maintained their RMR and fat-free mass, a.k.a. muscle tissue. Remember, we don't just want to lose weight; we want to lose fat, not muscle. The Weekday Diet group did just that, plus they maintained their RMR, meaning their bodies' use of calories remained efficient. This is huge!

I love this concept because it allows you to have some fun and extra calories over the weekend as long as you are good during the week. Basically, you buckle down during the week so you can enjoy some pizza or adult beverages over the weekend without any guilt. Heck, you should even feel good about it because you're ultimately getting better results that way!

Here's how The Weekday Diet can work for you:

- Eat one gram of protein per pound of body weight every day (even on the weekends).
- Do resistance training three to four times per week.
- Monday through Friday, fuel yourself at 35 percent below your maintenance calories.
- Saturday and Sunday, eat your maintenance calorie amount by increasing your carbohydrates.
- Do this for eight weeks, and see how you feel.

Here's an example to help; you just have to plug in your own numbers.

Let's say you are a cis male and have a TDEE maintenance level of 2,700 calories per day. During the week, fuel yourself with 35 percent of that, which is 1,755 calories per day. On the weekend, increase your carbs so you eat 2,700 calories per day. That would be an extra 945 calories of carbs, which would be about 236 more grams, which could look like three potatoes and three beers. Or six beers, I'm not judging!

Or let's say you are a cis female and your TDEE maintenance is 2,200 calories per day. During the week, fuel yourself with 35 percent of that, which is 1,430 calories per day. On the weekend, increase your carbs so you eat 2,200 calories per day. That would be an extra 770 calories, which would be about 192

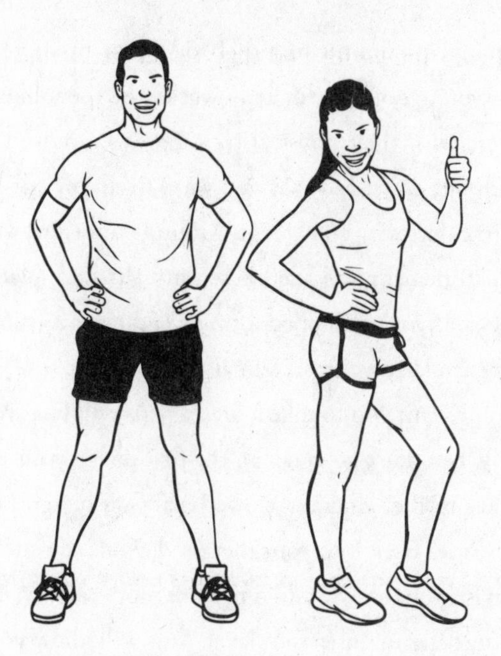

grams, which could look like three glasses of rosé and a large slice of pizza. See, I told you that you'd like this diet!

TAKE DIET BREAKS

No matter what route you decide to take—The Weekday Diet or the standard 10 percent calorie cut—I don't want you to be on a diet forever. Why? Because diets can make people go batshit crazy! Tell me if this sounds familiar. You start a diet and think, "Oh yeah, I got this!" You tell your friends, post on social media, and annoy the hell out of your family about how you are changing your life for the better. After a couple of weeks, you start getting a little bored, but you keep on because you're happy with the results. Then around week six, seven, or eight you basically turn into the spawn of Satan. You are hungry, hangry, sluggish, and just want it to be over. You eventually fall off the wagon, binge for several days, and then feel like crap that you ruined all your hard work. Been there? Don't worry, it's a common story, and one I've seen a lot.

Instead of trying to commit to a diet for a year or six months or forever, here's what I want you to do. Diet for eight weeks and then take a break. Athletes do this all the time with their physical training. It's a proven strategy. So why don't we do it with our diets? Let's say you want to simply cut calories. For your first week, cut your calories by 10 percent. Around your third week, consider cutting another 5 to 10 percent and stay there until the scale plateaus. During the last couple of weeks, if you've stopped losing weight, maybe cut another 5 to 10 percent. Remember to keep your protein at the same level the whole time. Once you hit week eight, I want you to take a break. This will help you both emotionally and physically. But don't go crazy on the first day of your break.

When it comes to diet changes, slower is always better. So start by adding 5 percent more calories back into your diet on day one. Be sure to eat foods you know will agree with you. Slowly add 5 percent more calories each day until you get back to your starting maintenance level. This will allow your metabolism to adapt, and you won't pack on a bunch of fat because your body was used to eating fewer calories and then you flooded it with a bunch of ice cream and chips. Enjoy this break for two weeks and then go back to your diet. When you return to diet mode, first calculate your new BMR and TDEE based on your new weight and then cut 5 to 15 percent at a pace that is reasonable for you. Heads up that you might gain a little weight doing this, but it will most likely be all water weight.

Which brings me to another important point—how much weight can you really gain in a short period of time? When people are concerned about gaining weight, they're typically referring to gaining fat. Most people wouldn't be opposed to simply gaining more muscle by going off their diet! But take the holidays, for example, or a vacation where you can't help but overfuel. Too often I hear people complain about gaining five or more pounds in a day. Um, no, you didn't. The scale may have said you gained 5 pounds, but that is not fat. It's mostly extra water and glycogen.

I'll share an interesting study to put you at ease. Researchers had people eat 1,000 extra calories per day for seven days.[32] The extra calories came from nothing but whipping cream, which is mostly milk fat. The study group was also super lazy and didn't train at all. This means they consumed 7,000 calories over their maintenance level. The results? They gained about 2 pounds. And of the 2 pounds, only one pound was fat, whereas the other pound was lean mass, which includes water and glycogen. Remember, they didn't work out at all, and their extra calories were not from nutrient-dense foods. They only gained one pound of fat in a week of eating 7,000 extra calories!! Imagine if they had been working out or if the extra calories came from whole foods. The results would have been much different.

The point is not to freak out if you eat over your normal levels for a day or two (or even a week). Your fat gains will be tiny. Going by the one pound people gained during a week at the 7,000 surplus, if you overfuel by 1,000 calories one day, you might gain 0.14 percent of a pound of fat. But that's if you don't work out. What if you used those extra calories to fuel your training and made it a heavy lifting day or intense cardio? Then those extra calories would be beneficial. So if you take a lot of calories in, just pay attention to your calories out.

WHEN & HOW TO PUT THE FORK DOWN

A common objection to following any kind of diet or eating plan is, "But I get really hungry." The truth is that maybe you're not as hungry as you think you are. How do you really know when you're thirsty, hungry, full, or satisfied? This is something a lot people struggle with, and the answer is both simple and complex.

If you normally eat at a certain time of day, then your body is programmed on a hormonal level to release ghrelin, the hunger hormone (think: *Grrrr, I'm hungry!*), around that time every day. That's why when people first start experimenting with fasting, they're ready to eat their own hands about an hour after their normal meal time. So the question is are they really hungry or is it simply the ghrelin telling them it's time to eat? In this scenario, it is most likely just the ghrelin talking. So here's my advice for trying any kind of fasting. Start by pushing your meals back by forty-five minutes each day. That's the sweet spot to delay the release of ghrelin. If you normally eat breakfast at 8:00 AM, push it to 8:45 AM for the first day or two, then 9:30 AM for a day or two, and so on until you get to your desired fasting window. Maybe it's twelve hours, fourteen, sixteen . . . Experiment until you find what makes you feel the best.

Now that you know this fun little ghrelin fact, how can you assess your hunger feelings and figure out if you're really hungry or if it's just your ghrelin talking? One trick is to drink mineral water or a glass of water with electrolytes. Sometimes it's simply a lack of trace minerals that will cause you to feel hungry. There are nine trace minerals: chromium, copper, fluoride, iodine, iron, manganese, molybdenum, selenium, and zinc.

Somewhere along the way, we were all convinced that salt is bad for us. But salt makes everything taste better so we all switched to sea salt because we were told it was healthier. Here's the thing, though—most sea salt does not contain iodine. And iodine is a mineral we all need, especially for the thyroid, which regulates metabolic rate, and helps heart rate, muscles, and digestion.

Go check your sea salt container right now. I bet on the front it says something along the lines of, "Does not contain iodine, a necessary nutrient." The truth is that salt is not your enemy. In fact, if you eat primarily whole foods and work out, salt can actually help with cravings, poor sleep, headaches, dizziness, energy levels, and recovery. So stop avoiding salt and go buy some iodized salt. FYI, you can find iodized sea salt. You can also find iodine in the following foods:

(RDA for iodine is 150 micrograms for an adult and 220–290 micrograms for pregnant and breastfeeding women.)

- Dried seaweed: I know, sounds weird, but I eat this monthly. A lot of companies now make flavored dried seaweed. It has a nice crunch and one-quarter of an ounce gives you 4,500 micrograms of iodine.
- Eggs: One of the most complete nutrient powerhouses, eggs give you 24 micrograms per egg.
- Shellfish: Lobster has 100 micrograms and shrimp has 35 micrograms. Most marine life whether an animal or plant will have iodine.

Get a weekly serving or two of fish for healthy fats and your iodine hit for that day.

- Cranberries and cranberry juice: This is my favorite. Just 4 ounces of cranberries have 400 micrograms of iodine, so ⅓–½ cup organic unsweetened cranberry juice (read the label; a lot of cranberry juice is crap) a day should have you covered.

Speaking of key nutrients missing from most diets—selenium is another big one. It's a trace mineral that helps the thyroid function properly and decreases oxidative stress.[33] The RDA for selenium is 55 micrograms for adults, 60 micrograms for pregnant women, and 70 micrograms for lactating women.[34] Most people aren't getting that, and it's really quite easy. Eat just one Brazil nut per day, and you'll get about 96 micrograms of selenium.[35] Other sources of selenium include organ meats, yellowfin tuna, and lentils.

After you drink that glass of water, wait fifteen minutes. If your hunger goes away, you weren't actually hungry. But if your stomach is still churning and asking for food, then you are legit hungry, and you should eat.

Okay, but what about the flip side of that coin—how can you tell when you're full so you don't overeat? Before I answer that, I want to share the hunger scale with you. I'm not sure who originally came up with this scale—I know it wasn't me—so I can't give credit where credit is due. To the original developer of the hunger scale—thank you!

Here it is:

1. Starving: You are literally a weak monster needing to crawl for your food.
2. Uncomfortably hungry: Your hunger is making it hard to focus on anything else.
3. Very hungry: You are ready to eat.
4. Slightly hungry: You could eat, but don't feel it's life or death.
5. Not full but not really that hungry: You are thinking about things other than food.

6. Satisfied: You could chow down more, but you don't need to.
7. Comfortable but a little full.
8. Very full: You are getting to that unbuckling the pants stage.
9. Too full: You are starting to feel bloated and uncomfortable.
10. Stuffed beyond moving: You are holiday full, feeling ready to go into a sleep coma.

So how do you use this scale? When you are hungry, you do not want to wait until you're at level one or two before you eat because you will likely overeat. Instead, eat when you are around a level three or four. This will help ensure you eat enough but not too much. Then you want to stop eating when you reach level six or seven. If you are eating mindfully—as I hope you will be—then you can tell yourself to put your fork down and give your body time to realize that you're no longer hungry.

The goal is to never starve or stuff yourself. You want to stay within the range of level three and seven. The order in which you eat your food can help with this. I recommend eating your veggies and protein first and saving your carbs for last. Veggies are full of fiber and protein is filling. Save your fruit for last as nature's natural dessert.

When you eat past level seven, you are getting into overeating or binge eating territory. There's a big difference between the two. Overeating is simply eating past feeling full to a level of eight or nine. Binge eating is when something almost takes over and you eat way past level ten.

One question I often get is whether overeating or binge eating can cause the stomach to expand, making it continuously easier to eat more and more. This is another one of those tricky questions that has two answers—yes and no. When you eat a lot of food, yes, your stomach is forced to expand to accommodate it. But once the food starts going through the digestion process and empties out, your stomach returns to normal size. This is why it's important to eat consciously, pay attention to how you feel, and stop eating when you start to feel full but still comfortable, per the hunger scale above. If you consistently overfuel past the point of comfort, you will get used to that feeling and continuously overeat. Overeating will become your new normal.

One last note about knowing when you're full. Remember, the goal is to always opt for whole foods first. They have the best chance of filling you up quickly so you don't overeat. Prioritize the following to help you fill up on healthy whole foods and keep you from overindulging on empty, crappy calories:

- Protein: Keeps your hunger hormone, ghrelin, at bay and is the most filling macronutrient.
- Fiber: Adds volume to food and slows the stomach-emptying and digestion time, allowing more nutrients to be absorbed and keeping you feeling full longer.
- High in volume: Foods that contain a lot of water and air, not a lot of calories. Think green vegetables and fruits. You'll never get fat eating spinach, kale, or watermelon, which is—wait for it—99 percent water!

STOP THE SNACKING MADNESS

Unless you are a competitive athlete or looking to cut down for a fitness show, it really doesn't matter how many times you fuel up in a day. That whole eat six to seven times a day thing was based on the thermic effect of food, meaning you burn calories by way of simply digesting macronutrients. This is true but it doesn't matter whether you eat six meals a day or three. Most people do not need to fuel up every hour or couple of hours. You see, the body has its own gut housekeeping system called the migrating motor complex (MMC).

The MMC is designed to clean your system by moving undigested matter out of your gut, keeping you regular and preventing infections such as SIBO. It takes your gut housekeeper anywhere from one to four hours to finish cleaning. But here's the catch—it only starts the gut-cleaning process when you are finished eating. That's why you want to space out your meals every three to four hours—so your MMC has time to fully clean your gut. And here's another catch.

Your gut housekeeper hates stress. That's why it's so important to relax, slow down, and prepare your body for digestion. If you eat in a stressed rush, your elevated cortisol levels will basically lock out your MMC, and your gut won't get any cleaning after that meal. So stop snacking so much and do a quick breathing exercise or meditate before you eat.

Your gut housekeeper also gets to work while you sleep at night, and that should be a nice, long cleaning window. In fact, don't be afraid to give your MMC even more time for overnight cleaning. Ideally, you want to go at least twelve hours between dinner and breakfast the next morning. But if you want to go longer and try a sixteen-hour fast with an eight-hour eating window, that's great. Because here's the thing. Breakfast isn't actually the most important meal of the day. That being said, if you turn into an angry warlock with headaches and mood swings if you don't eat within an hour of waking up, then by all means eat breakfast. Again, it comes down to knowing your body and finding what works best for you (do I sound like a broken record yet?).

MINIMUM METHOD FAVORITE FOODS

Here's the good news—there's a lot of delicious and nutritious foods to choose from. But that can also be bad news, as figuring out what to eat can be overwhelming, especially when you first change your diet. Don't worry, I've got you covered. What follows is a list of some of my favorite foods that I often recommend to clients. They're divided up into five main categories: protein, fats, carbs, vegetables, and fruits (plus I added extras). And yes, I realize that fruits can technically be considered carbs, but I like to classify fruits in their own category because of all the nutrients they have. Notice I have protein options for both meat eaters and nonmeat eaters. I believe people can survive and thrive on a number of different eating patterns, but overall, adding more plants to your diet will help you get the nutrients and fiber you need for a healthy body and microbiome. If you load your shopping cart with these foods and make them the mainstay of your meals, you will have a hard time not being healthy!

Protein

- Legumes: Beans, peas, and lentils are amazing sources of fiber and protein. These can be a mainstay of any dish or added as a nice side.
- Protein powder: You can do a lot with protein powder. In addition to adding it to smoothies, you can add it to Greek yogurt mousse—yum! Good sources of protein powder are whey isolate or a plant-based powder, which also adds a healthy amount of much needed greens. Another good protein source that has shown healing and joint properties is a collagen protein powder. This is inexpensive and can even be added to coffee in the morning in a fasted state. Look for collagen peptides for better absorption. You may be thinking that this is processed and therefore not a whole food. Ah yes, my smart reader. But this is one of those supplements that if it comes from clean sources and doesn't have a bunch of added sugar, it can be a great addition to your eating plan.
- Greek yogurt: For all you dairy lovers, Greek yogurt is critical. It has an incredibly high amount of protein and digestive enzymes, and it's low-carb. People with lactose intolerance can often handle Greek yogurt better than other dairy sources.
- Seeds: I've been adding hemp seeds to my oats and smoothies for years now. These nutty little seeds are loaded with protein, fiber, magnesium, iron, and healthy fats. I'm also a fan of pumpkin seeds for adding some crunch, protein (about 8 grams per ¼ cup), almost half of the RDA of magnesium, and good levels of niacin and zinc. Sunflower seeds provide protein (¼ cup gives you about 8 grams) and also has the all-important selenium. You can add flaxseeds to almost any dish for fiber, antioxidants, omega-3 fats, cancer-fighting properties, and about 4 grams of protein per 2 tablespoons. Try to have chia seeds daily for protein (2 tablespoons give you about 5 grams), omega-3 fats, about 10 grams of

fiber, and micronutrients. They're great in smoothies and overnight oats (made by leaving oats in a fridge overnight soaking in nut milk with maybe some protein powder added to it—so good!).

- Meat: I am actually fine with you having red meat, organ meats, and eating the skin of animals such as chickens. Red meat provides a ton of nutrients like B vitamins, zinc, and creatine. Organ meat is probably the best source of nutrition from an animal that you can get.
- Seafood: We don't eat enough fish nowadays. I want you to try to get one to two servings of fish per week for healthy fats, iron, zinc, magnesium, and potassium. Tiny fish, such as sardines and anchovies, are also powerhouses and have less mercury in them. Remember, the bigger the fish, the more mercury accumulation it has since it eats the smaller fish.
- Eggs (and eggs white): Yes, eat the yolks, but know that the whites have the most protein. These are true miracles in a shell. An egg is one of the most bioavailable sources of protein on the planet, meaning the body uses all of it. Eggs have choline for the liver to process fat, folate, zinc, calcium, phosphorus, B vitamins, vitamins A, D, and E, and eggs raise your good cholesterol (HDL).

First off, your body makes its own cholesterol. In fact, 85 percent of the cholesterol in your blood is manufactured by the liver, not the food you eat.[36] Cholesterol seems to be more linked to your family than anything else. But what about dietary cholesterol being bad? Well, for 70 percent of the population, eating cholesterol does not raise their bad cholesterol levels. But the remaining 30 percent of the population are hyper responders, whose cholesterol could increase slightly from eating eggs and other high-cholesterol sources.[37] What about cholesterol should you really be worried about? Trans fats! These are fats that are often labeled hydrogenated or partially hydrogenated vegetable oil. These will cause you all sorts of problems, including an increase in cholesterol.

Fats

- Wild-caught salmon and other fatty fish: Most people aren't getting enough healthy fats with omega-3 per week. You should consume one to two servings a week, and wild-caught (Pacific or Alaskan) salmon is a great source.
- Avocados: What's a shopping list without an avocado on it? I love replacing dishes that call for cheese or cream with avocado. The avocado has

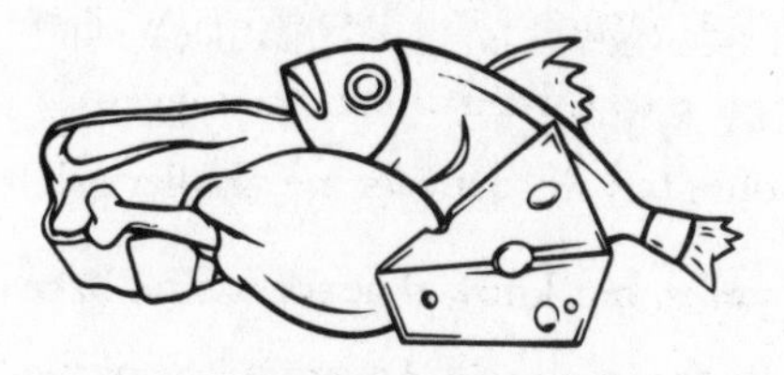

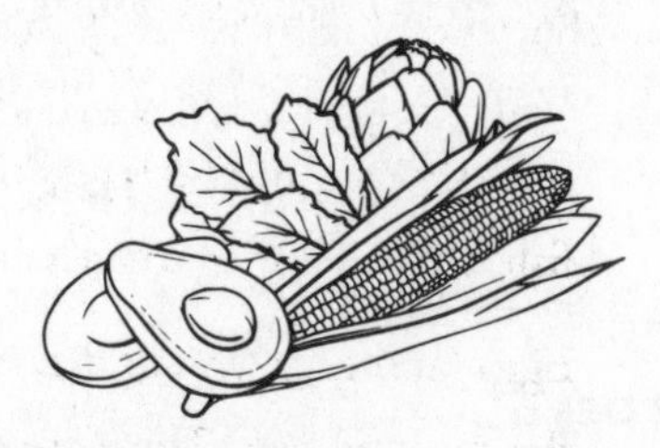

PROTEIN
PER 4OZ.

PROTEIN (PER 4OZ.)
BEEF: 30 GRAMS
BISON: 23 GRAMS
PORK: 23 GRAMS
LAMB: 23 GRAMS
CHICKEN THIGH: 20 GRAMS
SALMON: 23 GRAMS
HERRING: 14 GRAMS
COTTAGE CHEESE: 14 GRAMS
LOW-FAT CHEESE: 28 GRAMS
WHOLE EGGS: 16 GRAMS

PLANT-BASED PROTEIN
PER CUP

PLANT-BASED PROTEIN (PER CUP)
GREEN PEAS: 8.6 GRAMS
SPINACH: 5.2 GRAMS
CORN: 4.7 GRAMS
ASPARAGUS: 4.3 GRAMS
BRUSSELS SPROUTS: 4 GRAMS
ARTICHOKES: 4.8 GRAMS
AVOCADO: 4.6 GRAMS
KALE: 3.5 GRAMS
POTATOES: 3 GRAMS
MUSHROOMS: 4 GRAMS

fiber, potassium, vitamin E, and is pretty much the only keto-friendly fruit (important if keto is your thing).

- Nuts, assuming you don't have a nut allergy: Nuts provide healthy fats and have some protein in them, among other benefits. Remember, though, they are high in calories and fat, so if you are counting those calories, don't go nuts! Ha!
- Grass-fed butter and ghee: What? A book that says to use butter? Now don't go crazy with this as a little goes a long way. Get organic grass-fed butter or quality ghee. Both of these should be okay if you have a lactose issue. (Other great fats to cook with are avocado oil, coconut oil, olive oil (not in high heat), and bone or vegetable broths.)

Carbs

- Tigernuts: Get your stripes with tigernuts! They actually aren't nuts at all. They are tubers like potatoes and yams and have 10 grams of fiber and lots of potassium. Tigernuts are great for adding crunch to your meal or as a topping.
- Whole grains: Whole grains like quinoa, barley, farro, and spelt contain antioxidants, phytochemicals, fiber, and protein, and they really round out a meal!
- Baobab: This is an African superfruit that looks like a skinny watermelon on the outside and a pear on the inside. Baobab is great as a snack or smoothie addition because it's loaded with six times the vitamin C as an orange, and two times more calcium than milk.
- Black rice: This rice has an impressive amount of phytonutrients, vitamin E, and anthocyanins to help with heart disease. The only problem is it's hard to find. Yes, other forms of rice are acceptable as well. If trying to add as much muscle as possible and replenish glycogen stores post-training, then white rice is king.

- Potatoes (all kinds of potatoes and yams): Potatoes are filling and have a wide range of benefits. Those people who think potatoes are bad often associate them with how they are cooked or what's added to them. Remember, you can change the macronutrient profile of a food, making it fattier or higher in carbs, by how you cook it. If I bread and fry asparagus in seed oils, well, that doesn't resemble what it was in its original state as far as macronutrients and benefits.
- Bread: Another *what*? Yes, bread isn't entirely bad for you. Do I think you should have some crappy white bread or bread that is colored to look healthy? Of course not. But there are some good bread options that have a good amount of nutrients. Breads that I like are sprouted spelt bread because it's high in fiber and nutrients (not gluten-free), rye bread because it has three times less gluten than wheat bread so it may be okay if you have a gluten issue but not celiac, and sourdough bread (most are gluten-free, but read the label) because it is fermented so it's often more easily digested.

Veggies

- Greens, greens, and more greens: If it's leafy and green, put it in your belly! A study by The Produce for Better Health Foundation showed that most Americans aren't getting even one serving of fruits or vegetables a day. That's crazy! Pack your cart with fresh or frozen greens (amazing for smoothies) like spinach and collards. Greens can improve the digestion and nutrient absorption of your food, increase calcium, help your bones, and much more.
- Cruciferous vegetables: I'm talking broccoli, microgreens, and brussels sprouts, to name a few. They are packed with vitamins A, C, K, E, and B.
- Freekeh: Not only is it fun to say, but this roasted nutty green contains 10 grams of fiber (almost half the RDA) and 10 grams of protein. You can throw freekeh into many dishes that call for a grain such as rice or quinoa.

- Microgreens and sprouts: Both of these are young versions of their grown selves, such as broccoli, kale, and radishes. Sprouts are seedlings that are ready to harvest seven to ten days from sprouting, and microgreens are immature forms of their larger selves, ranging in size from 5 to 10 centimeters. Both should be added to a weekly diet, if possible, because they are loaded with benefits. Sprouts have a high antioxidant capacity due to the levels of polyphenols and L-ascorbic acid, as well as being superior to microgreens as a source of amino acids and pectins. But microgreens are high in chlorophylls, organic acid, and have high antidiabetic effects.[38] Try sprouts of broccoli, radishes, and lentils, and microgreens of radishes, amaranth, and kale.

Fruits

- Blueberries (fresh or frozen): These little guys are loaded with phytochemicals, soluble fiber, flavonoids, and antioxidants. A must for any shopping list. Also any other berry is a great option.
- Citrus from oranges to lemons: Of course they have vitamin C but they're also an excellent source of soluble fiber and flavonoids. Go ahead and munch away.
- Dragon fruit: This fancy-looking fruit is delicious and loaded with vitamin C and magnesium. It's also very social media worthy!
- You know what, while I'm at it, I'm just going to say any fruit: Most of us eat regular candy instead of nature's candy, which is fruit. Switch it up by season and enjoy!

Extras

- Organic coffee: Yes, I said it! Coffee can be an amazing source of antioxidants, can provide that caffeine kick, and has been linked to longevity.

- Apple cider vinegar: I use this on my salads, have it before a high-carb meal, and often use it for some extra flavor in my water. ACV can help with digestion for people with low stomach acid and even has blood sugar–lowering properties.

DIVERSITY MATTERS

In a perfect world, I would have you eating a massive variety of foods every day. But let's be honest—that's not realistic. So instead, I want you to try to cycle your foods and focus on switching up the five main categories: protein, fats, carbs, vegetables, and fruits. What do I mean by *cycle*? It can take a lot of forms, and I want you to find a way that works for you. While it would be great to cycle your food daily, let's be honest—that's probably not realistic. What is likely more realistic is grocery cycling, meaning just switch your foods up every time you grocery shop. If you have your grocery app dialed in to the point where you just hit Reorder every time, I don't want to mess up your rhythm. Just try to switch up one or two items each time you order. And I recommend everyone check out their local farmers market at least once a month to get some fresh seasonal foods. If you cycle the five main food categories, you'll reap the benefits of a high amount of gut diversity, get a wide array of nutrients without having to pop a bunch of pills, and enjoy quality complete protein even if you're vegan. Cycling will also create some nice variety in your meals so you don't get bored.

DON'T PANIC, CHOOSE ORGANIC

Okay, now remember we're going back to our roots and eating real food. Food that the earth naturally provides us like meat, vegetables, apples, nuts, and seeds. This is the food we were designed to eat. The problem is that through mass production, much of the way that food is grown has been tainted. So when you can, choose organic.

If you're not able to always eat organic, try to avoid the dirty dozen, twelve foods the Environmental Working Group lists as having the highest amounts of pesticides, herbicides, and fungicides, which when eaten can mess with our genetics.

These are the dirty dozen:

1. Strawberries
2. Spinach
3. Kale
4. Nectarines
5. Apples
6. Grapes
7. Peaches
8. Cherries
9. Pears
10. Tomatoes
11. Celery
12. Potatoes

And to make it a dirty baker's dozen, add hot peppers. If you're going to buy these foods, get organic as much as possible.

What about food that isn't grown but born? Here's the hierarchy when shopping for meat:

1. Organic, grass fed and grass finished
2. Organic and grass fed
3. Organic
4. Antibiotic-free
5. Pasture raised
6. Cage-free
7. Hormone-free

SUPPLEMENTS

Even if you fuel and nourish yourself with the healthiest foods on the planet, you can still benefit from the following supplements:

- Green powders: I feel most people should be taking green powders every single day with water or in a smoothie. They simply provide a ton of nutrients, fruits, and veggies that most people aren't getting. Try one serving a day.
- Chlorella: This green algae has a lot of chlorophyll, which gives green plants their color, and it has a lot of health properties.[39] But to be honest, the powder tastes like a mix of ass and dirt (if I knew what that tasted like). This is why I opt for the tablets. Chlorella has antiaging and antioxidant properties and has been used for deodorant, wound healing, blood building, energy, hormone balance, and even for cancer research. You can also choose spirulina, which has similar benefits.
- Multivitamins: Vitamin supplements are important to help fill the gaps of vitamins you are likely missing from your food.
- Vitamin D_3: This helps with calcium absorption, so without it, we can't have nice teeth and bones or proper muscle contraction.
- Omega-3 fats from fish oil: Omega-3 helps with a ton of bodily functions[40] such as inflammation, fat utilization, brain health[41] (lower risk of Alzheimer's[42]), and energy.[43] You can also get omega-3 from alpha-linoleic acid (ALA), which comes from plant sources such as walnuts, flaxseeds, or chia seeds.

MINIMUM METHOD EATING PROTOCOLS

Let's Go!

- Remove processed food from your diet. Nourish yourself with foods that have lived before. That means they have grown before, moved before, or swam before. Remember, real food doesn't have ingredients or a marketing company. Real food is the ingredients.

- Do not fuel up two to three hours before bed. This is not because of fat accumulation but because it will mess with your circadian rhythm while you sleep.
- Eat when you are calm and not in a hurry. Focus on appreciating your food.
- While you eat, focus on chewing your food slowly.

Level Up!

- Determine your BMR and how many calories you should fuel up with daily.
- Focus on your protein intake. Aim for getting around 1 gram of protein per pound of bodyweight.
- Nourish yourself with ten servings per day of vegetables, including leafy greens. What is a serving? If it is raw, it is about a cup or the size of your fist. If it is cooked (like cooked spinach or kale), it will cook down to about half the size of your fist. (If you can't get ten servings, eat more!)
- Have two to three servings of fruits per day. Eat berries as often as possible because they have the highest antioxidants, which are needed to fight free radicals, unstable atoms that can cause a host of issues to our cells linked to aging and disease.
- Eat carbs that only come from unprocessed sources like quinoa, farro, potatoes, and oats.
- Your fats should come from nuts, seeds, avocados, and limited oils.
- Fuel up three times a day with at least twelve hours between your first meal and your last meal the evening before.

- Do not eat until you are full; eat until you are just short of being full.
- Experiment with mindful eating strategies and stick to what works for you.
- If you have gut issues, consider doing the Thirty-Day Belly Bounce Back or a modified version.

Max Out!

- Try to fast for twelve to sixteen hours each day.
- Cook with avocado oil, ghee, water, or bone broth.
- Try to fuel up with greens and protein first before any high-carb meal as it limits the blood sugar response.
- Experiment with The Weekday Diet.

6

EXERCISE

Train Smarter, Not Harder

The majority of my adult life has been in fitness, and I used to think that's all that mattered. But as you should know by reading the chapters before this one, exercise is just one piece of the jigsaw. I truly believe—and research shows—that physical activity and being conscious of your movements are the best things for your overall health. But, as I've apologized for in the preface of this book, the fitness industry has lied to you. A lot. You don't need to "crush it" every time you train. You don't need to lift seven days a week. And you certainly don't need to do any crazy cardio. There is a time and place for those activities, but it is beyond the scope of this book and really beyond what most people need. Use this chapter as a guide and follow as many of the recommendations as you can, but also realize that I can't answer every single question you may have. In most cases, you can use your common sense. And yes, I'm going to again implore that you read the whole chapter, but—again—there is a lovely little CliffsNotes list of Minimum Method exercise protocols at the end.

When you go into a gym, your home, or outside to do cardio, I want you to exercise with intent. Think about why you are there and go in with a purpose and a plan. Do not go in without an idea of what you are going to do. Do you do that in business meetings? Likely not or you would be fired. So, for example, when it's an upper day, I want you to have a plan, be intentional, and focus on good form during every rep. Keep the reason you're exercising at the forefront of your mind so you get that added dopamine hit!

HOW MUCH EXERCISE DO WE NEED?

Being in the fitness industry for more than sixteen years, I spent a lot of time subscribing to the no pain, no gain mantra. I used to push my clients in every single training session. I even did it to myself. I remember times I couldn't walk right for days, had trouble sitting down on the toilet after leg day, or was unable to lift my arms to wash my hair after an upper body session.

My level of soreness became an indicator of how successful I thought my training was. The same thing happened to my clients. They used to get concerned if they weren't sore, worrying they weren't going to see results. Did a lack of soreness mean the training was useless? Of course not. But it's natural to ask that question when so much of the fitness industry is telling you otherwise. No pain, no gain, remember. Maybe we should say too much pain will limit our gains!

I'm not saying being sore is bad or that there isn't a time and place for very intense training. When FOX called me to train Terrence Howard to get him in "prison shape" for his role in *Empire*, you better believe he had many days feeling sore. We hit it hard twice a day for months and seriously dialed in his nutrition, sleep, and supplements. But keep in mind that was all part of the job. He was getting paid to look a certain way on screen, and I was getting paid to make that happen. It was a job for him, not a sustainable lifestyle.

Most of us have jobs that don't require ripped abs. We need to be able to function in our daily lives. That means you need to be able to walk up a flight of stairs in an office building or sit on a toilet without bracing yourself on the way down while cursing my name because you're so sore. Unless you're a movie star training for a role, you need to start with a training program that is realistic, functional, and sustainable for the long term.

In 2015, the *New York Times* published a blog post entitled "The Right Dose of Exercise for a Longer Life"[1] based off a *JAMA Internal Medicine* article that pooled data from six studies on the association between exercise and mortality.[2] The first study found that people who did not exercise at all faced the highest risk of an early death (shocking, I know!). Those who worked out a little (fewer than 150 minutes per week) reduced their risk of premature death by 20 percent. Individuals who worked out doing moderate exercise for the recommended 150 minutes or more per week had a 31 percent lower risk of dying prematurely. And the largest benefit came to those who moderately exercised—mostly by walking—for 450 minutes per week (about sixty-four minutes per day). This group had 39 percent less risk of a premature death.

A second study in the article looked at the intensity level of exercise. This is where it gets interesting. The people who spent 30 percent of their weekly exercise routine doing high-intensity activities such as interval training, rigorous cardio, or weight training were 9 percent less likely to die prematurely than people who did moderate-intensity activities for the same amount of time. People who spent more than 30 percent of their exercise time on vigorous activity saw a 13 percent decrease in mortality rate over the moderate-exercise group.

So what do these studies show? Do they prove the more-is-better scenario since people who exercised the longest per week and opted for higher intensity had the lowest risk of death? It may seem that way at first glance, but let's dig into it further.

Reading the study at face value has you walking away with a goal of working out for an hour every day with at least 30 percent of the workouts being high intensity. I'm going to point out another way to look at this. No one says your hour of training has to be in one session. Why not break up the time and spread your workout throughout your day? Maybe you don't have an hour in the morning, but I bet you have ten minutes.

MAKE IT SHORT BUT SWEET

In my experience, the biggest barrier to people hitting their fitness goals is lack of time. This idea of exercise snacking, or short bursts of exercise throughout the day can grant those who live busy lives in the real world a chance to get their 150 minutes in.

Research is starting to look into the impact of short bouts of physical activity throughout the day instead of longer durations of exercise at one time. Turns out, exercise snacking may be more beneficial in the long term. Taking a ten-minute walk after you eat has been shown to have insulin-controlling effects similar to that of the most popular prescribed diabetes drug, metformin.[3] Taking a ten-minute walk after three meals a day will not only control your blood sugar, but it will also stimulate your intestines and stomach to increase digestion, protect your GI tract, and even lower your risk of heart attack by lowering your LDL cholesterol (the bad cholesterol).

Another study out of George Washington University showed that older adults who took fifteen-minute walks about fifteen minutes after their meals at a moderate pace of 1,500 to 1,600 steps had significantly lowered blood glucose and HbA1c levels (another marker for glucose).[4] The walks were most effective at lowering blood glucose levels over twenty-four hours following an evening meal, which is often the largest. These results were just as effective as going for a forty-five-minute walk before breakfast.

Furthermore, doing a short but intense seven-minute training session (including a one-minute cooldown) before a meal has been shown to lower blood sugar concentrations within twenty-four hours more than doing thirty minutes of continuous exercise before a meal.[5] These short bouts can include an uphill walk, jog, or some kind of resistance training like push-ups or squats.

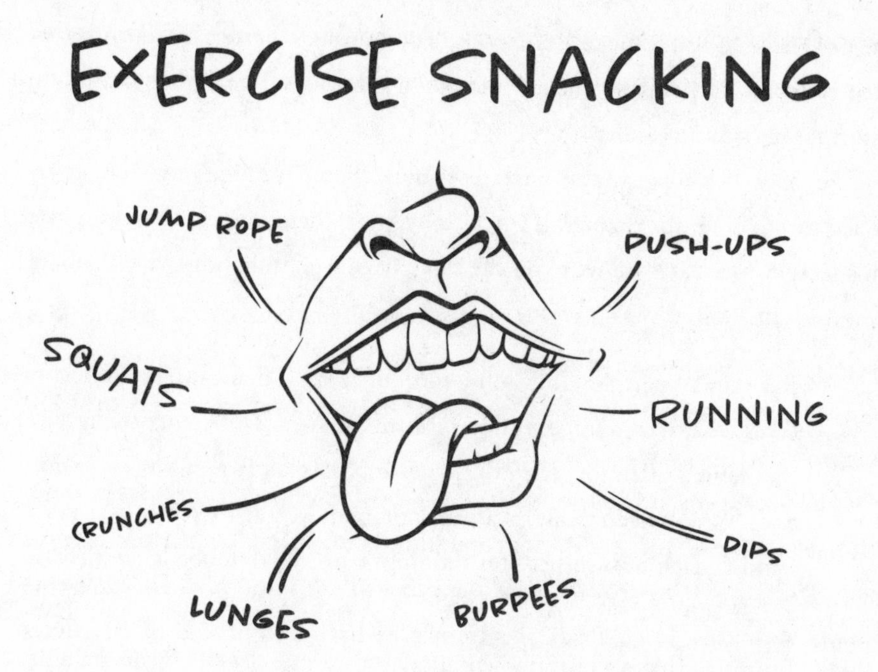

You might be thinking that a good workout requires a breakdown in muscle tissue for more muscle to be built, which means feeling sore. Sure, there is some truth to that statement. But the body adapts, repairs, and grows whenever it is exposed to a new stimulus and has been shown to increase strength and muscle size without damaging markers.[6] Starting any kind of new exercise plan can elicit results and gains just because it is new. There will be a time and place for longer training for performance and aesthetic reasons, and we will get into that a little later.

BACK TO BASICS

Most people aren't exercising effectively or efficiently. And that doesn't mean you need to start doing some crazy, complicated workout. Those big gyms can be intimidating. I get that. Luckily there are now a ton of at-home training and equipment options. Heck, you can start with zero equipment and simply focus on walking after you eat and doing some bodyweight exercises. At some point, you will need to add some resistance with bands, cables, or weights, but the first step is to break out of your mental and physical laziness. Remember, minimum effort for maximum results.

So, how should you train? First, let's go over some training terms I'm going to use throughout this chapter. If you already know these, you can just skim over this section to make sure we're on the same page regarding how we talk about working out.

- Resistance training: This is any form of exercise that causes a muscle to contract against a force with some form of external resistance to produce the desired effect of strength, hypertrophy (muscle growth), or endurance. Resistance training can include bodyweight exercises, resistance bands, machines, suspension training, barbells, dumbbells, kettlebells, and backpacks.
- Burning: This is a burning sensation in your muscles when you are resistance training or doing intense cardio exercises. Burning is nothing to be concerned about. When your body feels the burn, it is breaking down adenosine triphosphate (ATP) for energy, and hydrogen ions are being released. When there is a lack of oxygen in tissue (as it's being used while working out), you can't keep making hydrogen ions. This creates an acidic environment (not a bad thing), causing muscles to burn.
- Cardio: Short for *cardiorespiratory* or *cardiovascular* exercise. Cardio simply refers to any form of exercise that elevates the heart rate to pump oxygen and nutrients in the blood to the working muscles. A common misconception is that only standard cardio, like running or biking, is considered cardio. But any form of exercise, including resistance training and circuit training, can elevate heart rate and therefore be cardio. I mean, it's not like you stop breathing when you are lifting weights!
- Core training: Core training is often thought of as simply doing abs. But the core encompasses all the large and small muscles and fibers of the abs, lower back, and—I would argue—even the muscles above and

below, such as those in the hips, glutes, and lats. So I prefer the word *trunk*, as it is more encompassing. Your trunk keeps you upright, stabilized, moving, twisting, absorbing, bracing, balanced, and a lot more.

- HIIT: High-intensity interval training is a loose phrase that has been bastardized by a lot of fitness professionals and classes. True HIIT is meant to go from periods of high-intensity effort to periods of complete rest or active rest such as walking. The heart rate goes up for a period of time and then has an opportunity to go down for a period of time to recover. The original HIIT protocols called for a longer rest-to-work ratio as opposed to most that you see nowadays, where the rest is less than the work.
- Muscle confusion: A phrase that is simply referring to the periodization model developed by Soviet Union scientists who figured out that the body can physiologically respond and adapt to periods of high intensity (high stress) followed by low intensity (low stress). Here's what it does not mean—that you need to change your exercises up every time you train or you won't see results.
- Aerobic fitness (a.k.a. VO_2 max): VO_2 max is a large marker of your physical fitness. Essentially, it is the rate of oxygen consumption during exercises that are exhaustive, which can be resistance training or cardio. When you increase your aerobic fitness (or your VO_2 max), your body can deliver more oxygen to the muscles that are working, allowing them to work longer with less effort.
- Sets and reps: These are simply the number of times you do an exercise. For example, if you do ten squats, then rest or move on to another exercise, then do another ten squats, then rest or do another exercise, then do a final ten squats, you did three sets of squats at ten reps each.
- Isometrics: These are some of my favorite exercises and you have likely done them before, whether you realize it or not. Have you ever done a plank or a wall sit? How about holding groceries with a flexed arm?

Isometrics is when a muscle or group of muscles is activated and contracted without a change in the joints they cross. Think of it like flexing your arm and not moving it while holding a weight or a child (if you are a parent you know what I mean). Isometrics help with muscular endurance and are much better than dynamic exercises in terms of strengthening the spine and stability. This makes them amazing not only for sculpting that hot bod and sport-specific movements, but in rehabilitation settings as well.[7]

- Failure: The word *failure* gets a bad rap in most aspects of life, but in resistance training, failure is a good thing. The common definition of *failure* is when you reach a point that you can no longer do a single additional rep of a certain exercise. Your muscles simply say, "Nope, not happening." But I have a different definition of *failure.* When I say to do an exercise to failure, I mean to do it to form failure.

  When any movement starts to get really tough, people often change their form to get in those last couple of reps. Think using your body weight to swing those last couple of curls up. That's a no-no. When you can no longer do a single rep in proper form, that's when you reach failure.
- Rate of perceived exertion (RPE): RPE is how hard you perceive an exercise to be. Did the last several reps seem incredibly hard? Then you are at a 10 RPE.
- Reps in reserve (RIR): I prefer using this term, as RPE is more subjective. Most people don't know what a true 10 RPE feels like. But RIR makes more sense as most people can tell if they can get one or two more reps in before failing.

WHEN TO FEEL THE BURN

Let's talk about feeling the burn. Doing an exercise until you start to feel a burning sensation in your muscles is not a bad thing. It's basically a delay mechanism to help your muscles keep working. But you can overdo it. Some of the more-is-better propaganda in the fitness industry may have you thinking that every exercise in your training should get you to that burning point. If not, you didn't go hard enough. Please listen to me—that is not true! You don't want every set to get your muscles to burn, and they won't really burn until they experience enough demand on them. In fact, you should shoot for only about a quarter of your training to go to that point (unless you are an extremely experienced lifter). Why? Because the word *burnout* is legit. The burning sensation you feel is literally increasing the heat in your muscles, and they will eventually shut down. Employing the one-quarter method allows for better recovery times and joint health. So shoot for feeling the burn in only about one-fourth of your sets. This goes for cardio, too.

HIIT VS. MICT

There's a lot of debate about the best route to take to get to your goals. HIIT vs. MICT is a common argument. MICT doesn't get near the attention that HIIT does, yet it's probably done more often. MICT stands for moderate-intensity continuous training of less than 80 percent peak heart rate or aerobic capacity. Think going for a slow run, a long walk, and going on a hike. Basically anything slow and steady. Remember the tortoise and the hare? Well, HIIT (which in this instance is also classified as interval training or sprint training at efforts greater than 80 percent peak heart rate or aerobic capacity with bouts of short, intense effort followed by rests of lower intensities or complete rest) is the hare and MICT is the tortoise. When it comes to achieving better body composition, slow and steady can do the trick as well as being the hare—you can even sprinkle in some of both.

I'm going to share an interesting study with you, but I do not want you to latch on to it and use it as an excuse not to do one or the other. Too often, people see one study that reinforces their own wants, needs, or beliefs and then completely disregard any evidence to the contrary. A large meta-analysis compared

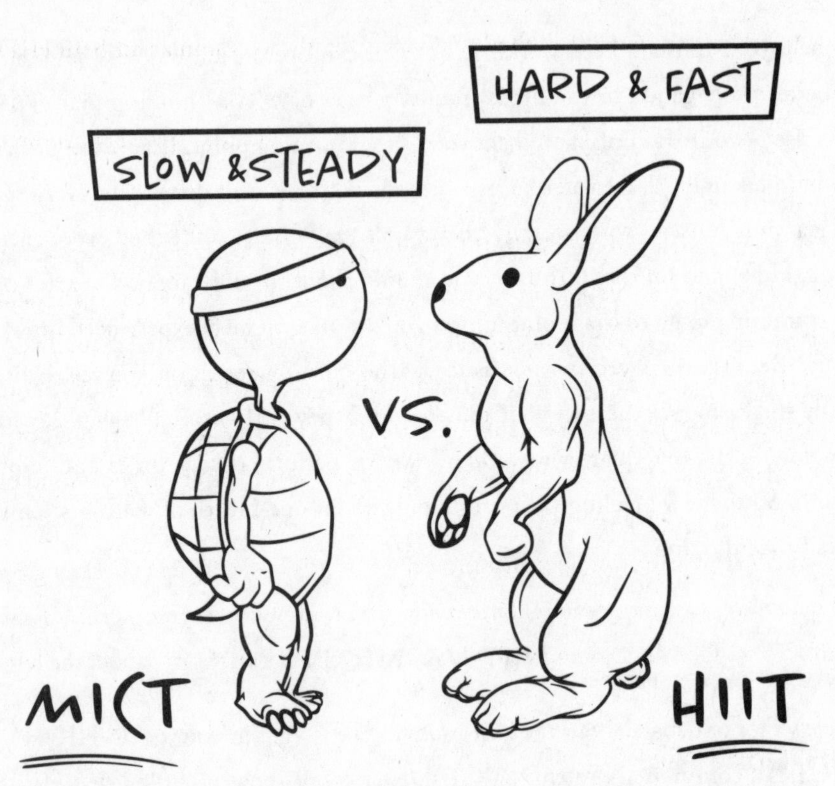

- HIIT AND MICT WERE ALMOST EXACTLY THE SAME WHEN COMPARING FAT-FREE MASS GAINS (EVERYTHING BESIDES FAT) AND FAT LOSS (CLOSE TO 1 LB)

- THE ADHERENCE (LIKELIHOOD TO DO ONE CONSISTENTLY) WAS SIMILAR.

- THE RESULTS OF HIIT HAPPENED IN HALF THE AMOUNT OF TIME BUT REQUIRED MORE EFFORT.

- WHEN IT COMES TO FAT LOSS PICK WHAT'S BEST FOR YOU. *ALTHOUGH THERE ARE POTENTIALLY MORE BENEFITS TO HIIT BESIDES BODY COMP FOR THE BODY.

HIIT to MICT in terms of body composition, losing fat while gaining or maintaining muscle.[8] Here's what it found:

- HIIT and MICT are equally effective in losing the same amount of fat (without diet intervention) over a twelve-week period, about 1 pound.
- HIIT and MICT are equally effective in gaining fat-free mass, like muscle.

- The adherence (likelihood to do consistently) was similar for both HIIT and MICT.
- HIIT achieved results in about half the amount of time but required more effort than MICT.

What does this all mean? HIIT might get you to your body composition goals faster, but it also might be harder to stick to. MICT is often easier for people to handle. My recommendation is always to do whatever you'll actually do. But HIIT has some other benefits, like mitochondrial health and working more fast-twitch muscle fibers (fibers that produce a lot of power and energy but don't have a ton of endurance), so I like to see people do some sprints or some kind of HIIT at least once a week.

The bigger point is it doesn't really matter what you do, so don't get hung up on semantics. Just move more. If you enjoy HIIT, go for it. If you prefer MICT, then do that. Do whatever you will actually stick to, and don't worry about the rest.

HIIT Done Right

As I mentioned above, a lot of HIIT training today isn't structured properly. Trainers and HIIT classes are not allowing for enough rest time in between the high-intensity intervals (if that's good news to you, you're welcome!). This is yet another example of the fitness industry constantly pushing the more-is-better agenda. Take a sprinter, for example. They may sprint 100 yards in ten seconds, but they're not going to turn around and do another sprint five to ten seconds later (and if they did, their time would be much worse).

To explain how to do HIIT training correctly, you need a quick lesson in biomechanics. When you first start performing any kind of exercise—no matter what the intensity is—your body relies on your quick energy system to start moving. This system is called the adenosine triphosphate phosphocreatine system, or ATP-PC. It only lasts for ten to fifteen seconds of maximum effort and then your body needs to switch to another source of energy. So when you're in a fitness class and you're told to sprint for a minute, that's technically impossible. You can run as fast as you can for a minute, but you only have ten to fifteen seconds of ATP-PC stored before it needs a break to replenish. But that's really just semantics.

Here's how true HIIT is supposed to work. For every second of work, you need ten to twelve seconds of rest for recovery. The work can take on many forms, including running and sprinting, biking, doing high knees, lifting a really heavy weight for a rep or two, and punching a heavy bag. It can even be walking fast and then walking slowly or walking up a hill and then down a hill. Remember, exercise intensity is relative. A true interval is a period of work followed by a period of rest. And not just thirty seconds of rest; enough rest that you can recover.

The problem with most of today's HIIT classes is that they don't give enough rest, and they're too long. You don't need to do HIIT for an hour. Sure, you get a good sweat and you're out of breath and it feels hard so you think you had a good workout. But it's not necessarily good for your system. Can you see results with HIIT? Sure, at first. You'll burn a lot of calories, but you won't maximize your results in any one particular area. Form usually goes to shit during a HIIT class, and there isn't enough symmetry (anterior vs. posterior) in the training. You will likely see results when you first start doing it, but your body will adapt and you'll quickly plateau. Beginners will most likely overtrain because they don't need to train as much to get results. So here's my official stance on HIIT classes—they may have a place in your overall training routine, but doing them all the time will stress your body too much.

If you want to do HIIT, here's a good one. This seven-minute workout was developed by researchers to maintain muscle and strength in the shortest amount of time possible. To do it, simply perform all the exercises listed below for thirty seconds each, with a ten-second rest in between each exercise. The goal is to do them as quickly and as safely as possible (except for the isometric holds).

- Jumping jack, burpees, or high knees
- Wall sits or simply squat and hold it
- Push-ups (on or off knees or a bench) or clapping push-ups

- Crunches (not sit-ups) or leg lifts
- Bench or chair step-ups or split jumps
- Squats or squat jumps
- Tricep dips or narrow push-ups
- Plank or mountain climbers
- Lunges forward or back or to the side
- Jump rope, sprint, high knees, or hill run
- Push-ups with a rotation or up-down plank (high to low plank)
- Side plank or fire hydrant

CLARIFYING MUSCLE CONFUSION

Here's a fact—you can get great results doing the same exercises for weeks on end. Even months! I would even argue it's better to do the same exercise routine because it gives you a standard for your training—you know exactly what to do, and you know when you're ready for more.

The concept of muscle confusion comes into play when your body has adapted to what you've been doing. Only then do you need to worry about modifying your training to "confuse" your muscles. But this doesn't mean the exercises have to change. Any small change will work, whether it's lifting a little heavier or changing your tempo. Here's an example.

Let's say you want to be able to do more pull-ups. To get stronger so you can do more pull-ups, you don't need to be jumping around from yoga to Pilates to some crazy HIIT class to build the strength you need (though yes, doing other back-resistance exercises and building synergist muscles that work together to create a movement will help). You simply need to keep doing pull-ups. Your body needs consistency with a certain type of stressor to adapt, grow, and get stronger.

Generally speaking, you can be on the same program for four weeks to several months as long as you stick with the concept of progressive overload, meaning you add more weight when you can. It doesn't need to be large weight increases. Think 2 to 5 percent each week or every other week. Decreasing your tempo or even doing more reps with a lighter weight can also do the trick.

If you're worried about getting bored doing the same workout all the time, then you can switch up the movements so you're hitting the same muscle group at different angles. For example, maybe you do curls with dumbbells one day and curls with cables the next. It's a similar motion but slightly different angle and stimulus, allowing you to switch up your exercise but keep the intensity and volume consistent so that you build strength. Another way to change the stimuli but keep your exercises the same is by simply changing the weight used (intensity) and the volume (sets × reps), a concept called nonlinear periodization. Let's say you're doing a three-day-a-week, full-body training program, which is amazing for everyone from beginners to advanced lifters. You can make one of those days your heavy day, where your reps are in the four to eight range. Make the next day a medium-intensity day, where you do eight to twelve reps. And the final day can be a higher-volume day with reps at twelve to twenty per exercise. Studies have shown this type of training is effective for both strength and fitness gains.[9]

WHAT ABOUT CARDIO CONFUSION?

Okay, so we know we don't need to be constantly switching up our strength-training routines, but what about cardio? Should you stick to your usual cardio routine or should you change things up? Remember, anything that elevates your heart rate can count as cardio. Well, almost anything—a scary movie doesn't count, but a little nooky (wink wink) does!

Whether or not you need to spice up your cardio depends on your reason for doing it. What do you want to get out of your cardio? Are you doing it for weight loss, general health, specific athletic goals, or because it's good for your mind? If you run a couple of times a week because it helps to clear your mind, then I say to keep at it as long as you're also getting some resistance training in.

I will never advise someone to stop doing cardio if it helps them mentally, even if they're trying to gain as much muscle as possible. Never devalue the benefit of a strong mind. If you're running for an athletic goal—like a race—then you're going to have to do the same form of cardio (running!) for weeks on end, and that's fine. But if you are doing cardio for weight loss or aesthetic goals, then I recommend you do different forms of cardio or play around with sprints and intervals while running. This not only allows for some hormetic stress to create adaptation, but also allows you to work in different planes of motion, and focus on balance or speed.[10]

JUST GET FITT

Here's a good rule of thumb when trying to improve your exercise endurance, burn more calories, or lose fat. When you feel like you are hitting that plateau (and believe me it won't be after three to four weeks), it's time to change things up and get FITT. The FITT rule of thumb can be applied to cardio and strength training. FITT stands for frequency, intensity, time, and type:

- Frequency: If you are a beginner and have been working out one or two days a week, then add an extra day. Or if you are only doing my suggested ten-minute walks or the exercise snacking, add in another snack or walk, or, better yet, add a resistance-training day.
- Intensity: You can increase intensity with the number of sets or reps you do, or even with your heart rate training. For example, if you have been walking at 60 percent of your max heart rate, go the same distance in a shorter amount of time and try to increase your heart rate to 75 percent. These little minimum effort bouts can truly help! Don't know how to find your heart rate if you aren't wearing a tracker? Simply take your pulse on your blood vessels either on the inside of your wrist or on your neck outside your trachea. Count how many beats were in ten seconds and then multiple by six.
- Time (duration): Simply add an extra five minutes to your cardio sessions or your resistance-training sessions (don't go over an hour for resistance training).

- Type: Change the type of training completely. Instead of running, go for a swim. Instead of biking, do a resistance leg day. Instead of yoga, do Pilates. Instead of walking on a flat surface, walk up some stairs. I simply want you to move more and move consciously. What does moving consciously mean? It means you're aware and paying attention to your body—from how it's moving to how it feels.

INCREASING YOUR VO_2 MAX

Whether you're doing resistance training or cardio, your muscles need oxygen to function. Cue your VO_2 max. As I stated earlier, this is a huge indicator of your overall fitness level. When you first start exercising, it's pretty easy to increase your VO_2 max without even thinking about it. The key is pushing yourself outside your comfort zone, specifically when it comes to your heart rate. The more in shape you get, the more you'll have to proactively focus on pushing yourself to the point where you can increase your VO_2 max.

To improve your VO_2 max, you need to get your heart rate up to above 90 percent of your maximum heart rate and keep it there for at least a minute, ideally for three to five minutes. An easy way to calculate your maximum heart rate is to simply subtract your age from 220. I'll be thirty-nine years old when this book goes to print (likely forty by the time you read it, yikes!), so my max heart rate is 181. For me to improve my VO_2 max, I need to get my heart rate up to 163 beats per minute (181 × 93 percent) and sustain it there for several minutes. When you calculate yours, it might seem intimidating, and I get it. But you need to stress your body to create long-term changes for your health. That's why I went on my rant earlier about lazy cardio. I'm not asking you to sustain that high heart rate for twenty minutes. I just want you to push yourself to the point of discomfort, just for a little bit. Doing so will increase your VO_2 max, which will increase your life span, decrease your risk of stroke, improve your mood, and much more.[11]

Unfortunately, there is no good way to test your VO_2 max without the use of fancy equipment, but that doesn't mean you shouldn't work toward it either directly or indirectly. So, let's talk about how to put some VO_2 max work into practice. Any form of exercise that brings your heart rate close to your max can help, but here are some specific ways to work at it:

- Push yourself during a quarter of your training. The burn I talked about earlier can be felt in either your muscles or your lungs. No need to track it like a scientist here, just really push yourself one-fourth of the time.
- Interval training, whether it's true HIIT or today's definition of HIIT, is one of the best ways to increase your VO_2 max. It's been shown to be even better than steady cardio at a heightened heart rate.[12] I like intervals of hard work for thirty seconds to one minute followed by a one- to three-minute break. You can do this with traditional forms of cardio, like running or biking, or you can do it with bodyweight exercises or weights at a quick pace. Maybe squat as quickly as you can for thirty seconds and then take a thirty-second break and repeat that for five to ten minutes. There are a ton of ways to get there—just push yourself safely.
- Pace runs so you run fast (not all out) for one minute, then jog slowly for two minutes, then run as fast as you can (or sprint) for thirty seconds. Repeat that process several times. Remember, this is all relative. Your jog looks different from anyone else's and looks different than it did twenty years ago. Don't compare yourself to anyone else or to any time other than right now.
- I know dancing on a bike is all the rage right now, but I'm a big fan of biking for a purpose. Start with a nice, easy pace as a warm-up for ten to fifteen minutes. Then increase your speed (or tension or both) to the point where it's tough but you can still hold a conversation and continue for fifteen minutes. Then perform intervals going as fast as you can (add some tension) until your heart rate reaches that 90 percent mark, and try to maintain that for three to five minutes. Then you can slow it down for a few minutes and ramp it back up or do a ten-minute cooldown. During each ride, try to go a little longer or do an extra sprint. All in all, you're done in twenty-five to thirty minutes.

How long will it take to see changes in your VO_2? Well, research says you'll see improvements in as little as a month.[13] If you've already been training, you could see a 5 to 30 percent improvement in twenty weeks,[14] and likely even more if you haven't been working out.

DO THESE EXERCISES EVERY DAY

I don't want you to freak out and think you need to train seven days a week. You might get there at some point, but that's not what I'm about to suggest. Instead, the following moves are more like stretches to help with form when you do train and will result in overall better body posture and mechanics.

Brace for a Better Body

Bracing is very important for keeping proper posture, body alignment, injury prevention, and when lifting weights. Best part is it can pretty much be done anywhere any time. I'm doing it right now as I sit upright and type this section while also practicing my nostril breathing (read the breathing chapter if you haven't yet) with my laptop right at my eye level to help with my posture. No one wants text neck, a.k.a. upper crossed syndrome. I want you to practice and perfect bracing before you move on to anything else in this chapter. Bracing has been shown to work the deep abdominal and superficial muscles, help with gait while running to minimize pelvic motion, help with posture, and more.

Unfortunately, just like most of us aren't breathing correctly, most of us don't naturally brace either. You must learn how to do it and what it feels like before you can incorporate it into your daily life (and posture!). The following exercise is a great introduction to bracing. You get the feeling and control while lying down so when you finally practice while working out, you know the sensation and can better get that mind and muscle connection. Here's how to practice bracing:

1. Lie on your back on a firm surface.
2. Put your feet on the floor with bent knees.

3. Put your hands on your hips with your fingertips in front of your hip bones.
4. Take a deep breath in through your nose.
5. Slightly press into both sides of your abdomen with the tips of your fingers.
6. Now tighten your abs as if you were getting ready to take a punch.

Think of this as adding intra-abdominal pressure or an internal weight belt to provide a stiffening of the core. Once you get familiar with the feeling, you can start bracing throughout your day, particularly when sitting at a desk and when lifting heavy weights. If you are doing a heavy deadlift or squat, you want to inhale a lot (like 70 percent) and tighten your abs hard. But if you're only picking up a grocery bag, you don't need to be that extreme.

Bulletproof Your Back

About 80 percent of the population will have back pain one day. I've had several herniated disks from playing college hockey, so I'm already contributing to that upsetting statistic. Here's the funny thing about back pain—it's usually not really your back. More often, back pain is really stemming from another area in your body, namely your core. When I focus on the core, it is to get the parts of the body to work together as a unit, both when stationary and when moving.

The following three exercises will help strengthen your trunk, or core, and decrease your chances of back pain or issues. I promise these can be done every day and won't leave you sore or debilitated. They will only take a couple of minutes. I call them the Three to Be Free. Free from what? Free from all the issues you get from sitting too much, like tight hips and weak glutes, that will one day wreak havoc on your back if they haven't already. In my experience, 99 percent of people have some sort of lumbo-pelvic-hip dysfunction from sitting too long or an altered firing pattern with their body. Essentially your muscles don't fire or "turn on" in the correct order they should and one muscle will take over for the other that should be working. This could be something like the hamstring firing before the glutes when the glutes should be first in a movement such as the hip thrust. The Three to Be Free are all about mobility and addressing these issues, for if you have tight hips, a tight lower back, or weak glutes, doing normal core work, or any other work for that matter, could just exacerbate the problem. I recommend doing the Three to Be Free before any cardio and resistance training session, or just as a good reason to get up off your lazy ass.

Here are the Three to Be Free exercises (you can also find these at joeythurman.com/minimumtraining):

1. Hip flexor stretch: Hip flexors are often overactive and short, and they need to be lengthened. You can release the hip flexors with this stretch, which can be done either kneeling or standing. Bonus points if you can foam roll—using a large "rolling pin" type object that can be purchased online or at any sporting goods store for self-myofascial release (SMR), similar to a self-administered massage . . . just maybe a little more painful—your quads, hip pocket (think the crease above your front jean pocket, below the bone on the front side of your hip), and the large part of the front of your leg before doing this. Here's how to do it:

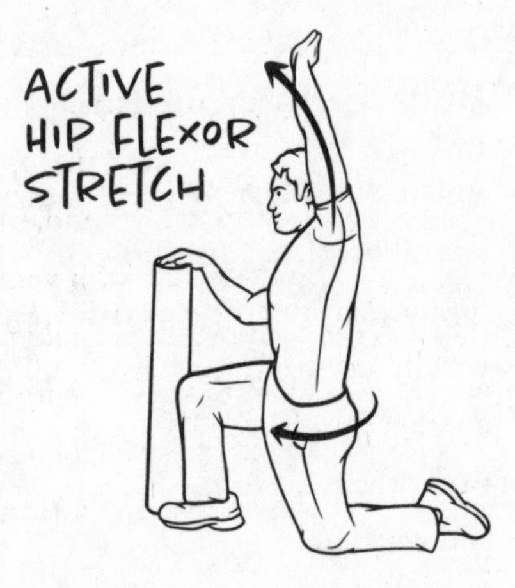

    1. Kneel on one knee with your knee directly beneath your hip.
    2. Straighten and lengthen your spine.
    3. Squeeze the glute of the leg with the knee on the ground (not with your hand, weirdo—with your mind!). This will start to release the hip flexors because of reciprocal inhibition, which means that when one side of a joint is activated, the opposing muscles are forced to relax.

4. Slightly shift your weight forward without overextending your back, and hold for thirty to sixty seconds.
5. Repeat on the other side.

2. Cat camel: This will help with mobility of the spine and relieve lower back stiffness without compromising the lower back like some other stretches do. Think spine-friendly mobility. Here's how to do it:

    1. Get down on all fours with your knees directly below your hips and your hands below your shoulders.
    2. Slowly arch your entire spine while lifting your hips as high as you can without any pain so that your back is in a rounded position. Your head should be looking down and you should look like a camel full of water (yes, their humps have water in them). Hold this for a few seconds.
    3. Then perform the opposite motion—push your chest and belly toward the ground, arching your back in the opposite direction, and look up with your head so you look like a cat in an extended position. This should feel like a nice, light stretch without any pain. Hold this position for a few seconds.
    4. Do five to seven rounds of this. Yes, only five to seven rounds, which should take about thirty seconds to one minute.

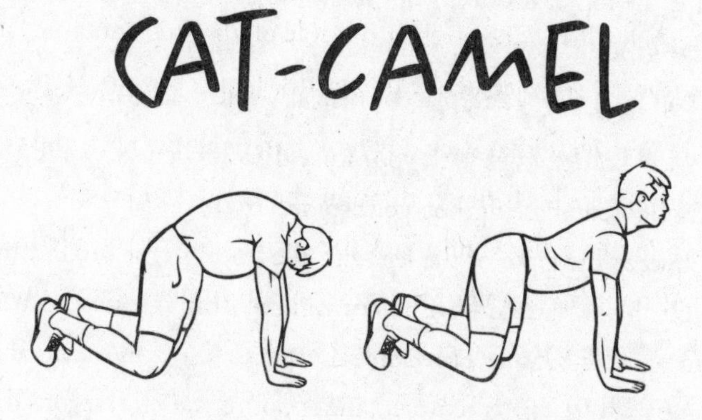

3. Towel Glute Bridge. Once your booty is all loose, it's time to activate it.[15] Don't confuse this move with a hip thrust. Hip thrusts are great, but they have more of a range of motion. The bridge is wonderful because it also works the deep cervical neck flexors, which are usually underactive because we are constantly looking down at our phones. We're starting to look like turtles on two feet, and that's not good. Forward head posture[16] is correlated with an increased risk of neck injury,[17] changes in muscle activity, upper thoracic flexion, loss of lordosis, and possible auditioning for the role of the Hunchback in the next Disney movie.

NECK/GLUTE BRIDGE

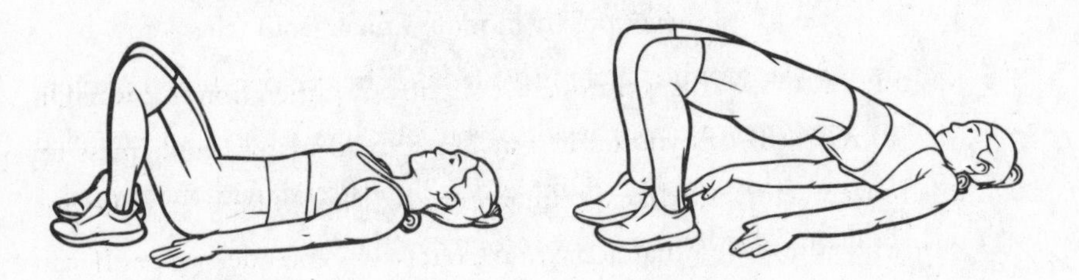

Here's how to properly do a towel glute bridge:

1. Lie on your back with your heels under your knees and feet flat on the ground. Your shins should be vertical.
2. Roll up a towel and place it beneath your neck. You want to think about driving that neck down to flatten out the neck and the towel.
3. Drive your heels down through the ground to bring your hips up while squeezing your glutes the entire time so you are in a bridge position. Be sure not to overextend the lumbar spine. Think maximum proper rep range and not excess.
4. Then slowly lower your hips—under control—and repeat for twenty to thirty reps.

Common overactive muscles that need to be released include the upper traps, levator scapulae, rhomboids, sternocleidomastoid, scalenes, and cervical extensors. Common underactive muscles that need to be activated are deep cervical flexors, serratus anterior, and lower and middle traps.

After you do the Three to Be Free, it's time for The Big Three. To give credit where credit is due, I modified these from the work of Dr. Stuart McGill, the world's leading practitioner on back health. I've swapped out one of the exercises he recommends with one I like better. The Big Three focus on the core to help protect the back, but you need mobility in order to do these moves. The Three to Be Free above will help loosen you up and activate the muscles needed to do the following exercises.

Here are The Big Three . . . kind of.

1. Modified curl up: This is the one I've slightly modified from the way Dr. McGill recommends you do it. But I've seen so many people mess up this move and treat it like a crunch because it looks and feels like one instead of the abdominal activation exercise it's intended to be. If you treat it like a crunch, you run the risk of overworking the psoas, which is the muscle connecting the lower back to the upper thigh deep in your abdomen to either side of your belly button.[18] Here's how to do it:

    1. Lie on your back with one knee bent while the other is straight.
    2. Place your hands underneath your lower back to keep the natural curve in your spine.
    3. Pick your head up off the ground just a few inches and hold that position for ten seconds. Lead with your chest, not your neck. Remember, this isn't a crunch, per se, but you will naturally have a flexed abdomen. If your head were on a scale, that scale would not measure a single pound. As you hold, try not to move your lower back, maintaining the same position you started with.

4. After the hold, bring your head back to the ground to reset at the starting position.

If you want to make this movement harder,[19] you can squeeze your abs before the head movement and only have your hands on the ground, and your elbows and forearms off the ground, creating less stability. Perform five reps on each side for ten seconds each. Then take a thirty-second breather and do three reps alternating sides for ten seconds each with a thirty-second breather, and then one set each side for ten seconds. This is called a descending pyramid.

2. Side plank: The side plank is a great exercise to work the lateral stabilizer of the oblique's (a.k.a. love handles), the quadratus lumborum (QL) muscle, and the gluteus medius, which helps stabilize the hip.[20] It can be done with the legs out or the knees bent to start. Here's how to do it:

    1. Lie on your side with your elbow below your shoulder and your feet outstretched.
    2. Take your top leg and put it in front of your bottom leg. Don't stack your legs, as that will create pressure on the lumbar spine.
    3. Lift up to bring your hips off the ground.
    4. Hold this for ten seconds, drop down, and do five sets of the side plank for ten seconds on one side and then switch.
    5. Take a thirty-second breather and repeat for three reps each side for ten seconds, rest, and then do one rep each side for ten seconds.

    To make this harder, you can hold it for longer, lift your front leg in the air over the planted leg, or even do some rotating side planks.

3. Cross crawl, or bear crawl. The original Big Three calls for the bird dog exercise as the third move. The bird dog is a great way to work overall core stability, so I recommend doing the same progressions outlined below. But I recommend doing a cross crawl (or bear crawl), as it is a great way to work the posterior oblique subsystem and train natural movement patterns. It works the stabilizers, reinforces a gait pattern,

and turns on the transverse abdominals. It's also hard to cheat on this one. Here's how to do it:

1. Get down on your hands and knees (all fours). Make sure your knees are below your hips, and your hands below your shoulders.
2. Flex your feet so your toes stay on the ground as you lift your knees about an inch or two off the ground. You should feel your abs activate. Hold this position for a few seconds to get used to it.
3. Then crawl by moving one arm out and your opposite knee in (think left arm out and right knee in). Then move the opposite limbs to crawl forward slightly.
4. Do five crawls forward and five backward. Take a breath.
5. Do three crawls forward and three backward. Take a breath.
6. Do one crawl forward and one backward.

If you do the Three to Be Free and the modified (or original) Big Three daily, you will have a strong core and a bulletproof back.

CHOOSE YOUR LIFTS WISELY

When it comes to lifting weights, there are several ways to skin a cat and different equipment that can be used. I love all sorts of different equipment, from machines to dumbbells, bands, kettlebells, medicine balls, and more. I don't want you to think of there being a "wrong" exercise, but instead there can be a wrong form or wrong execution based on your specific needs and goals. For example, an athlete who uses a lot of cutting motions and one leg stability may benefit more from doing a single leg movement that looks fancy, whereas you could simply do a squat or leg press. One isn't necessarily better than the other, just better for the situation.

Too often, the fitness industry tries to split hairs when it's not necessary. Some people may disagree with me, but all you really need to do is focus on the main movement patterns, which are push, pull, press, twist, hinge, squat, and loaded carry. Below is a list of exercises that use these movement patterns. By no means is this list exhaustive. Whether you want to put on muscle, lose fat, gain endurance, get stronger, or achieve a combination of these, you can choose from the list that follows to develop a program that will meet your goals. Don't focus only on what you want so you forget what you need. If you lack stability, be sure to do some balance work with single-leg moves. If you've been skipping one too many leg days, make sure you give yourself a few sets of legs each week.

For more exercises and to see video demonstrations of all of the below, head to joeythurman.com/minimumexercises.

THE MINIMUM METHOD LIFT GUIDE

Even if an exercise doesn't call for weights, you can always add them. Most of the exercises mentioned here can be done holding dumbbells, kettlebells, or back loaded (weights on your back like a bar). For step-by-step demonstrations of each, go to joeythurman.com/minimumexercises.

- **Glutes**
  - hip thrust
  - single-leg hip thrust
  - barbell hip thrust
  - glute biased squat
  - split squat
  - hip extension with cable or bands
  - dumbbell single-leg hip thrust
  - glute bridge

- banded glute bridge
- single-leg glute bridge
- walking lunge
- leg press
- Smith machine squat
- step-ups
- reverse lunge

▸ **Quads**

- barbell back squat
- dumbbell quad dominant squat
- leg extension
- dumbbell or kettlebell goblet squat
- leg press
- Bulgarian split squat
- high step-up
- reverse lunge
- front lunge
- side lunge
- b-stance squat

▸ **Hamstrings**

- hamstring machine curl
- stability ball curl, single-leg or both
- stiff-leg deadlift
- b-stance deadlift
- bodyweight single-leg deadlift
- glute ham raise

▸ **Upper Pushes**

- chest press
- push-up
- chest fly
- cable chest press

- — cable chest fly
- — incline chest press
- — bench press, any angle
- — neutral shoulder press
- — military shoulder press
- — barbell push press
- — chest dip
- — dumbbell shoulder press
- — banded shoulder press
- — banded chest press
- — banded chest fly

▸ **Upper Pulls**

- — bent-over barbell or dumbbell row
- — single-arm bench row
- — split stance row
- — cable machine row
- — lat pull down
- — pull-up variations
- — band row
- — band pull down

▸ **Rotations**

- — dumbbell wood chop
- — cable trunk rotation
- — medicine ball throw
- — twisting side plank
- — rotating lunge
- — transverse squat
- — landmine chop
- — cable low-to-high chop

▸ **Loaded Carries**

- — dumbbell or kettlebell farmer's carry
- — hex bar farmer's carry

- — single-arm farmer's carry
- — weighted bag or plate-hug carry
- — suitcase carry
- — Zercher carry
- — double kettlebell or dumbbell rack carry
- — overhead carry
- — overhead grapevine
- — bottoms-up kettlebell carry

▸ **Accessories**

- — plank variations
- — hollow hold
- — bear crawl
- — leg raise with posterior tilt
- — lateral crawl
- — lateral raise
- — triceps extension
- — triceps kickback
- — biceps curl
- — superman
- — IYT
- — pullover
- — dumbbell prone rear delt fly
- — standing cable or banded hip abduction
- — banded leg adduction
- — sled push or pull
- — calf raise
- — seated calf raise
- — wall toe raise for anterior tibialis
- — kettlebell swing

Now that you have a nice list to choose from, we can get into how you should be working out. Don't worry, I will cover cardio as well later in the chapter.

SOMETHING YOU KNEED TO KNOW

How many of you have heard—or been told at some point—not to let your knees go past your toes when squatting or lunging? It's become a common word of caution, and one I always thought was dumb. It's just another example of using one study out of context that said it could lead to knee pain and making it a general rule. Think about it. When you go to stand up, your knees go past your toes. When you walk up or down stairs, your knees go past your toes. It's a natural part of movement, not the villain it's made out to be. We need to train our bodies in all planes of motion.

Look down at your leg and straighten it out to make a muscle with your quad. Do you see that teardrop muscle above your knee toward the inside part of your leg? That is your vastus medialis (VMO), which is one of the four quadriceps muscles. Being so close to the knee, the VMO is a fast-twitch muscle, which means it reacts fast to protect the knee. Due to knee issues and lack of use, a lot of people don't have a great VMO. Training the VMO and other muscles and tendons that help the knee function will increase blood and nutrients in the area, make the tendons around the knee stronger, and bring additional synovial fluid around the joint to restore pain-free motion. Translation: it will make your knee healthier. One of the best ways to train the VMO is to walk backward. That's right, walk backward.

Remember, I want you to take a ten- to fifteen-minute walk after your meals. Well, why not make them backward walks. Don't worry, your neighbors and coworkers will eventually stop looking at you funny. When you walk backward, check out your knee relative to your toes—it's in front of your toes. That means it's working your knee and your VMO. Walking backward will actually help you walk forward better.

Walking backward is also a great warm-up before training. Or you can include more backward work within your training to make you more athletic, run faster, and jump higher. If that's your endgame, then follow the progressions below.

If you can, do these on your leg days or at least once a week to start.

1. Backward walk with a sled: Tie a rope to a sled and attach the other end to a belt around your waist. Walk backward pulling the sled.
2. Backward deadmill: A deadmill is when you walk or run on a treadmill with it turned off. So a backward deadmill is—you guessed it—walking or running backward on the treadmill when it is turned off.
3. Backward hill work: Walk, run, or even sprint backward up a hill. Don't go down the hill backward. Do that forward!

What's the answer to the knee-location debate while squatting and lunging? Here's my recommendation. If you have enough hip and ankle mobility (meaning your feet can stay flat on the ground while squatting), then there is no issue with your knees going past your toes. I have a long tibia and femur and a lot of mobility, so my knees often go past my toes. If you don't have enough ankle mobility, then you need to address that first. Start rolling out the bottom of your feet, calves, and lower leg, and then stretch. Even doing ankle rolls can help gain more mobility. Another tip is to use a wedge, book, or small weight plate below your heels when you squat or lunge to immediately give your ankles more dorsiflexion (backward bending of the foot so that the toes go toward the shin).

REP IT OUT

Let's get into the nitty-gritty. Knowing how to train is just as important as the moves that make up your workout routine. In this section, there are answers to some of the most common questions I get about training. But remember, above all else always listen to your body. What is best for your body will be different from what is best for your friend's, coworker's, or training partner's.

How Many Reps and Sets Should You Do?

This is an important question, and sadly the answer isn't cut-and-dry. Here is the thing—research is now pointing to a number of rep ranges that can help with fat loss and adding muscle tissue, or hypertrophy. The old adage "lift big to get big" has some truth, but you can also lift light and get tight (ooh, I like that!). My guess is that most of you reading this book aren't trying to be a powerlifter or go for records in weight lifting. You simply want to feel good and look good. There is a time and place to do heavy lifts (five reps or less of high energy) that prioritize getting strong by way of mechanical tension and adding muscle tissue. But for longevity purposes, you can be successful doing twenty-five or more reps as long as those last two to three reps are strenuous, and you don't feel like you could do twenty to thirty more. Effort and intensity matter.

According to the International Universities Strength and Conditioning Association standard on muscle hypertrophy, you can successfully add muscle tissue at a low load of high reps of fifteen or more, moderate load of reps between nine and fifteen, and high load at reps of eight or less. The general consensus on recommendation seems to be to stick primarily with a moderate load of six to twenty reps while every now and then using other loads. But you can mix it up however you want. The important thing is to be intentional and strategic in terms of your goals. An example of a lower body circuit I love is a high load of squats for six to eight reps, then a medium load of hip thrusts for nine to fifteen reps, and ending with a low load of cable hip abductors for a burnout round of fifteen or more reps.

Low load: A weight that allows you to do fifteen or more reps with good form and close to failure, or with one to two RIR.

Moderate load: A weight that allows you to do nine to fifteen reps, and you couldn't do one more rep with good form past fifteen.

High load: A weight that is close to your one-rep max and allows you to do only one to eight reps to failure, and you can't do one more with good form.

Do You Need to Train to Failure?

No. But the effort needs to be high. You can still see great results when you stop with one to four RIR or short of failure. There have been many studies looking at this,[21] and there are benefits, like better recovery, to not training to failure. Just make sure to push yourself and don't leave ten reps in the tank. That's not conducive to getting maximum results. As you become more trained, you may need to start pushing that pain threshold and going for all-out effort.

How Much Exercise Do You Need in a Week to Maintain Muscle?

As few as five sets per muscle group per week is all you need to maintain and possibly even see results.[22] It depends on factors such as your prior training volume, genetics, and diet. At a minimum, simply do a full-body workout to hit every muscle group for five sets of eight to twelve reps. You could do this all as one training session or split it into two. It doesn't take a lot, people!

Of course, your level of training matters. The good news is if you are a beginner, you can practically grow just by driving past a gym. Not really, but studies show as little as three sets of ten repetitions a week can increase strength and size in a new trainee. As time goes on, there is a diminishing return. But studies show that even well-trained cis men can see strength gains from a mere six to twelve repetitions with loads ranging from 70 to 85 percent of their one-rep max, done two to three times per week for eight to twelve weeks.[23] The key is high effort with momentary muscle failure.

Check out the chart on the next page.

Remember, this is a guide; it's not absolute. When you look at this and see twenty sets per week per muscle group, don't automatically think more is better. For some people who are highly trained, this may be the case. But most people will not benefit from that much exercise. Instead it will hinder their results.

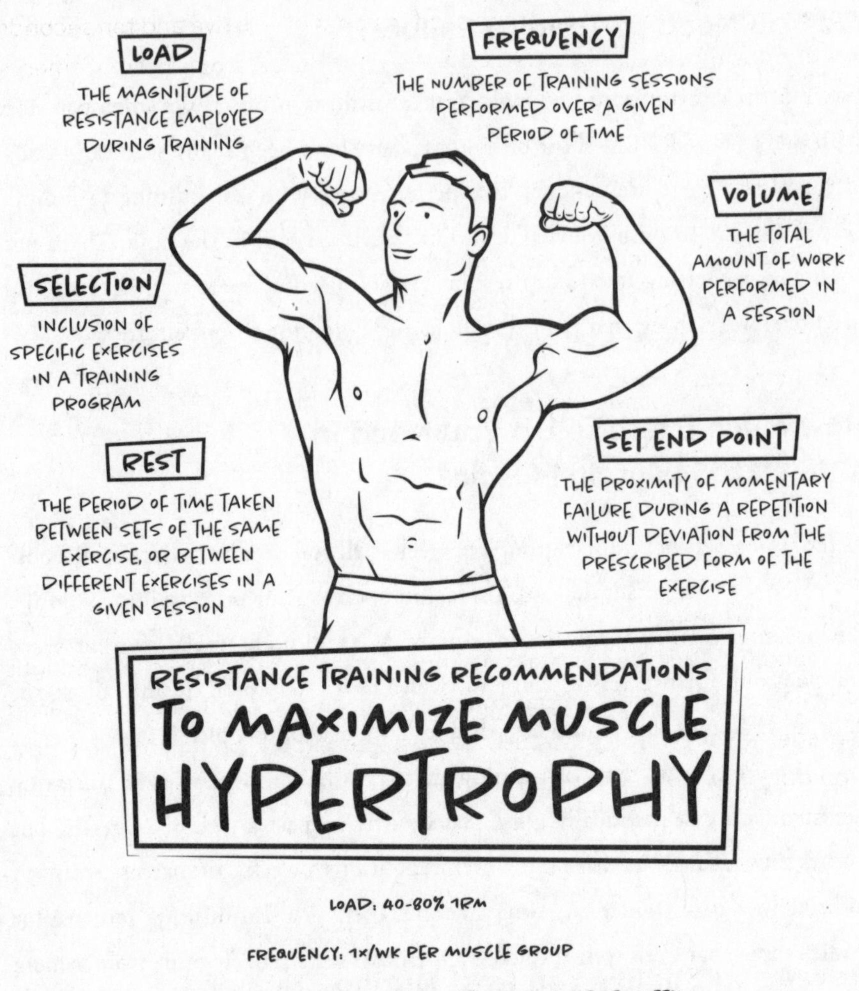

A lot of research looks at people who already train regularly, but what about those who don't or have taken decades off? Yes, if you played high school football thirty years ago and haven't lifted more than a beer since, then I would consider you a beginner. One of the largest studies of its kind looked at 14,690 people who worked out only once per week for about seven years.[24] Their one workout was supervised by a trainer, consisted of six different exercises, and lasted less than twenty minutes. The exercises were done at a super slow speed of ten seconds on the negative and ten seconds on the positive without locking out the joint on the pressing movements and not fully extending (or unloading) during the pulling movements. The exercises included chest press, lat pull down, leg press, abdominal flexion, back extension, and alternating days of hip abduction or adduction (typically performed in that order). Rep ranges were from four to six to the point of momentary muscle failure, increasing the weight as needed per session to stay within that range. So each set lasted from eighty seconds to two minutes. That is a long set with a high time under tension.

The results? Massive gains (30 to 50 percent) were made during the first year of this protocol, but they seemed to level off dramatically after year one. About six years later, using the exact protocol, gains were still improving, but only 50 to 60 percent from baseline. But they still got stronger doing the same exercises, simply increasing the weight when need be! You see, you don't always have to switch up your routine to gain or maintain strength.

This study also shows massive implications as we age. We are thought to lose about 1 percent of our muscle mass and strength each year after the age of thirty, but this study shows that simply doing this one slow workout once a week for less than twenty minutes can help us maintain our strength and muscle.[25]

How Long Should You Rest During Training?

If you're trying to maximize muscle growth or fat loss, you want to keep your rest periods relatively short. Think thirty to ninety seconds between sets.[26] Why? Because rest affects hormones.[27] Shorter rest maximizes the release of the hormones involved with muscle growth and fat loss. If your goals are more strength and power related, meaning less emphasis on how big your muscles are, you need more rest so your nervous system can recover enough to allow you to lift a higher load. Studies indicate that a two- to five-minute rest is best for strength and power.[28] Those rest ranges are pretty wide, I know. So here's some more guidance. You want to match your rest periods with your exercise. If you are performing a multi-joint exercise, like a squat, you will need more time to recover than if doing a single-joint exercise, such as a bicep curl.

However, if your goal is to maximize your calorie burn during your resistance training, then I want you to pay more attention to your breathing than the clock when it comes to rest. To burn more calories, you want to maximize your excess post-exercise oxygen consumption. You can do this with the talk method. Basically, your goal is to get out of breath to the point where you can't hold a conversation for the majority of your training. That could mean heavier loads or it could mean less rest time. Either one can get you above your aerobic threshold and cause your body to burn more calories for up to twenty-four hours after you train.

How Long Should Your Training Be?

There can be too much of a good thing. In general, you want to keep your resistance training to around forty-five minutes or less, no longer than an hour if you can help it. Working out for too long can elevate your cortisol levels and inflammatory pathways,[29] putting you into a catabolic state, which breaks down metabolism and can hinder your efforts in the gym.

Do You Have to Do Cardio?

If you hate cardio, I have good news for you. A large study showed that even one hour-long weight training session per week showed significant improvements in cardiovascular health, including a 40 to 70 percent decrease in risk of cardiovascular disease, 32 percent drop in risk of cholesterol issues, and 29 percent lower chance of developing metabolic syndrome.[30] Should you take this data and think you only need to train once a week? Well no, but you can start there at a minimum. Doing something is always better than doing nothing!

HOME GYM EQUIPMENT: THIS IS ALL YOU NEED

Not everyone wants to go to the gym, especially since COVID-19. I totally get that. That's why home gyms have become all the rage. But you don't need to go crazy with home gym equipment. I've put together a list of essentials for any home gym. Most of these are portable, which is important to me because I like to take them on business trips and vacations. And yes, I train while on vacation. There's nothing like working out in the sun while getting a tan! My wife often joins me, and to be honest, she totally outshines me. And I'm totally okay with that!

- Suspension strap that can be tied to any tree or pole (TRX is a popular brand).
- Kettlebell.
- Mini band (small-looped bands).
- Power band or resistance band.
- Jump rope.
- You! That's right, you are your own gym.

I also love working out while wearing a weighted vest.[31] Get one and wear it during your cardio, walks, or even while weight training for some extra resistance. Even if you don't resistance train (and you know you should by now), a weighted vest can help burn calories and enhance performance. Choose a vest that is 5 to 10 percent of your bodyweight.

Here's a list of some of the exercises that can be done with this equipment. A great training session is to choose six exercises and do them all for thirty seconds each, taking a fifteen- to thirty-second breather in between. Do that several times.

Step-by-step instructions for each exercise can be found at joeythurman .com/minimumtraining.

- Suspension strap: Rows, triceps extensions, split squats, mountain climbers, curls
- Kettlebell: Swings, bent-over rows, goblet squats, walking lunges, wood chops, presses
- Mini band: Three feet apart foot taps, monster walks, victory raises, banded squats
- Power band: curls, shoulder presses, lateral raises, chest presses, triceps extensions, squat presses
- Jump rope: Double hops, high knees, one foot
- Body weight: Push-ups, lunges, side lunges with rotation, bear crawls to the side or front to back, plank variations, mountain climbers, squat thrusts, skaters

CARDIO DONE CORRECTLY

First, a note on movement in general. Remember, our bodies adapt to what we're doing and can be efficient in conserving energy. We always need to be aware of that and adjust accordingly. When you start working out, whether it's resistance or cardio, your body will try to conserve energy in other areas of your life. I recommend you wear a step watch and always try to hit a certain number of steps per day to maintain that extra energy loss. This could be something as simple as five thousand steps on your training days (not including the workouts themselves) and ten thousand steps on your non-training days. You can easily reach this with the recommended ten-minute walks after your meals.

Okay, let's dive into cardio. I don't care what kind of cardio you're doing; I just want you to remember the three *m*'s. These are critical for cardio success.

1. Measure: Start at a baseline level that you know you can handle for a few weeks. Maybe it's running or maybe it's simply walking on a treadmill at an incline. Just be consistent for a couple of weeks to see how you feel and what results you are seeing.

2. Maximize: Then it's time to pick it up! Each week, increase your activity a little bit. That could mean going for longer, increasing your pace, or increasing your treadmill incline. Just keep increasing a little each week.
3. Maintain: Make sure you are in control of everything you are doing with your diet, resistance training, and steps to make sure you avoid compensating for your cardio. Once you have gotten to your desired weight, set a new goal for yourself and a program to get there. Don't lose the momentum!

Now let's talk about specific cardio recommendations.

How Much Cardio Do You Need?

As always, the answer depends on your goals. If you simply want to maintain cardiovascular fitness, you don't need to put a lot of time into it. An interesting study done on soccer players found they were able to maintain their VO_2 max simply by doing a twenty-minute HIIT session once every two weeks.[32] Here's what they did (and what you can do too):

- Four minutes of intense cardio (87 percent or more above your max heart rate or to the point where you can't maintain a conversation).
- Rest for four minutes or do some light recovery work like a plank or arm exercises.
- Repeat for five rounds/sets.

The entire training session takes thirty-six minutes. The exercise modality can be running outside or on a treadmill, biking, air boxing, jumping rope, swimming, or jumping jacks, among others. All that matters is that you do it at a high-effort level.

If your goals for your cardio are to build muscle endurance, you want to lean more toward a higher number of rounds/sets (fifteen or more) so the exercise is demanding on the muscular level as well as the cardio level.

Should You Eat Before Cardio?

From a fat-burning standpoint, it may be advantageous to do your morning cardio training fasted. A recent study in the *British Journal of Nutrition* shows that you can burn up to 20 percent more fat when doing cardio in the morning in a fasted state.[33] Why does this work? While you sleep, your body breaks down amino acids into glucose, so working out fasted in the morning mobilizes fat (especially if you have some black coffee, green tea, or yerba maté tea before) and potentially uses more amino acids as fuel while you're training. If you are trying to build muscle, this isn't ideal. But if you have a meal or protein shake post-training (ideally within an hour or two), you will be fine.

That being said, if you feel lightheaded and have less energy, then you should eat something. People often have more energy when they have food in their system. More energy means you work harder and therefore burn more calories and fat because you have food in your system. My advice is to do some training fasted and some not and see how you feel.

If you're strength training in a non-fasted state, consider doing some light cardio immediately afterward. Because strength training utilizes glucose as the main energy source, doing some light cardio afterward is like doing cardio in a fasted state and helps burn more calories and fat.

Tired of doing the same old cardio? I've got you covered. Remember being a kid and jumping on one of those mini trampolines or, better yet, the really big ones that you fell off of (okay, maybe that was just me)? A study done by the American Council on Exercise found that not only did jumping on a trampoline, or rebounder, mimic a moderate to vigorous intense workout, but it also produced the same benefits as running at a six mph pace, playing football, or cycling in only nineteen minutes, and likely with less joint issues.[34] Better yet, participants had lower perceived exhaustion, meaning they felt like they weren't working as hard.

THE MINIMUM METHOD COMPLETE 180

I created this exercise program years ago for an online competition. I didn't win—WTF?—but it's still a really great program. Now, it doesn't live solely in the resistance or cardio camp. It's more of a combination. This type of training is considered a metabolic conditioning workout. Translation: it gets your metabolism firing, your muscles burning, and your cardiovascular kicking! I named it the Complete 180 because you complete 180 reps as safely and as quickly as you possibly can. It can be done anywhere, any time, and by anyone. I recommend you do it one to three days a week (especially if you are strapped for time).

I want you to push yourself with this training. You will most likely be done in fifteen to twenty minutes. Have fun with it and keep track of your time so you can see if you can do it faster the next time. Get uncomfortable during this training to create change in your body and mind. Trust me, this fifteen minutes of discomfort is better than a lifetime of discomfort in your skin.

There are three different exercises. You can pick other exercises but these were specifically chosen because they challenge every muscle in the body as well as the cardiovascular system. This group of exercises makes for full-body training, but you can switch it up to focus only on the upper body, legs, core, and so on. Your tempo should be fast but under control. If you need to take a break at any point, take one. Once you've caught your breath, continue with the training.

Here's how it works:

Exercise 1: Scaption or T raise to get the upper and middle back.

Exercise 2: Reverse plank knee tuck to train your shoulders, back, and adductor muscles on the inside part of your legs.

Exercise 3: Squats or jump squats.

Round 1: Sixteen reps of each exercise. Rest

Round 2: Fourteen reps of each exercise. Rest.

Round 3: Twelve reps of each exercise. Rest.

Round 4: Ten reps of each exercise. Rest.

Round 5: Eight reps of each exercise. Rest.

This training session will leave you feeling accomplished, ready for the day, and exhausted!

CARDIO & RESISTANCE: TO COMBINE OR NOT TO COMBINE?

I hope by now you understand that you need both resistance training and cardio. Whether you make some of your resistance training a cardio workout as well or keep them separate, I don't care. But things can get a little tricky when combining cardio and resistance in the same session. Think going for a short run and then lifting. Without getting too sciencey, here's the thing. Resistance training activates certain pathways that are beneficial for your health. Doing too much cardio during a weight training session can shut down important pathways.

If you want to do both during the same session, here's what I want you to do. Perform light cardio before or after your weight training session, as it is not likely to block your gains. For any more serious cardio—like endurance training—separate it by doing cardio in the morning and your weights later in the day (at least four hours later). Or do it on different days altogether. But, as always, it comes down to your goals. If you want to gain as much muscle as possible, then you should cut your endurance training down to one to two times a week or even not at all.[35] But honestly, most people don't need to worry about this, as the amount of cardio you're doing isn't enough to hinder your gains.

THE EXERCISE BATTLE OF THE SEXES

There's a lot of talk about how gender impacts training styles and whether women and men should train the same or differently. Personally, I don't take gender into account when training anyone. I train based on goals. Now, people may have different body parts they want to target, but as far as overall training style, gender plays no role. Everyone is equally capable of gaining strength and putting on muscle.

That being said, cis women do have one thing that cis men do not, and that's a menstrual cycle, and I do take that into account when training cis women. Some phases of the cycle create more energy, whereas others make for less energy. Your cycle can also change your calorie needs. To me, it's asinine to expect a cis woman to train through a heavy flow day when she is losing a lot of blood and water and is likely weaker and therefore more prone to injury. It might seem odd to have a cis man telling you women about your menstrual cycle, but hear me out.

First, I recommend you start tracking your cycle, training, and how you feel during each phase. You can track this with an app, in your phone notes, or simply use good old pen and paper. A cis female cycle has four phases: menstrual, follicular, ovulatory, and luteal. There's a lot going on in your body and with your hormones at any phase of your cycle. Here are my recommendations for scheduling training around the different phases:

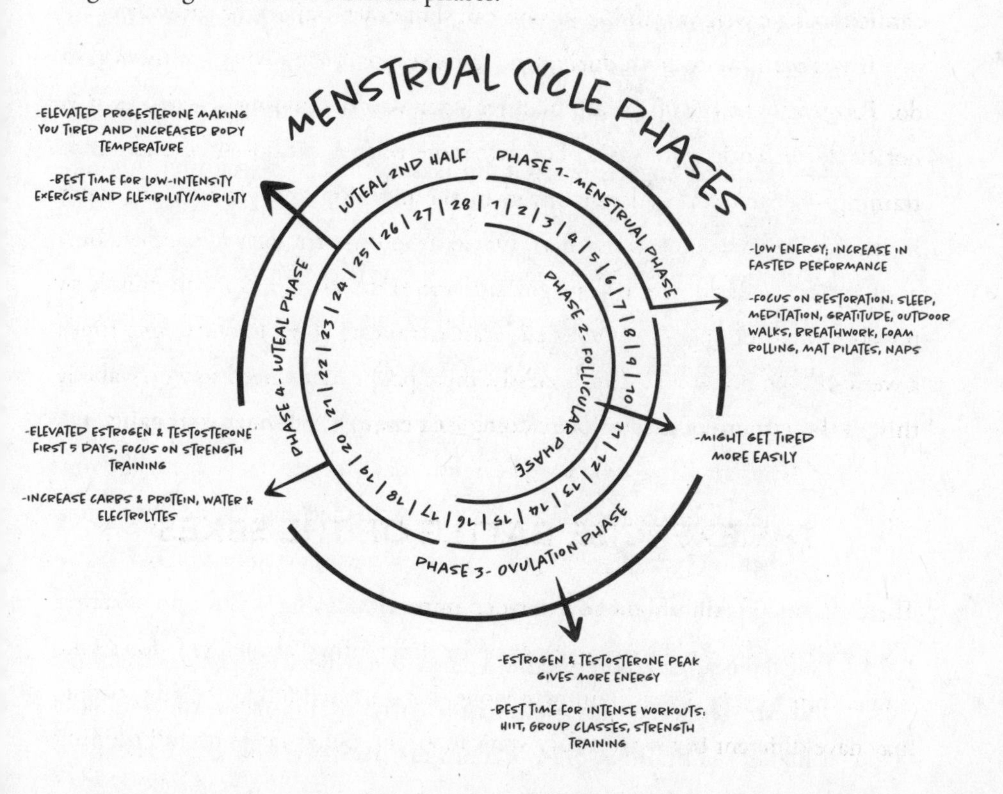

- Menstrual phase (about three to seven days): Hormone levels are at their lowest during this stage,[36] so you are likely to feel a little weaker. But the feelings of weakness won't actually inhibit your ability to gain strength. Going too hard during this phase of your cycle could cause you to become more tired and place stress on your cardiovascular system. This is the time to make sure you get your proper rest and sleep.
  - — Training suggestions: As you are likely to be more drained during this time, schedule more working-in exercises, like meditation, yoga, tai chi, breathwork, foam rolling, stretching, mobility, or light Pilates. If you are going to resistance train, be aware of the volume load and take longer breaks between exercises. Opt for shorter workouts during this phase. And it's probably not the time to HIIT it up!
- Follicular phase (about sixteen days): Once you have stopped bleeding, you might feel a sudden increase in energy and mood. This is a good time to try new things, as you are more welcoming to new people and experiences. You may even have an increase in willpower to avoid cravings for bad food, as your mood is enhanced due to the rise in estrogen.[37]
  - — Training suggestions: Group classes, resistance training, hiking, sprints, and rebounding.
- Ovulatory phase (three to four days): This is the phase when you have the highest levels of testosterone and estrogen. It's also when you're the horniest, and remember—sex counts as exercise!
  - — Training suggestions: This is the time to get after your training and push it. This could even be a time for two-a-days if you feel like you need to make up a day when you weren't feeling as good during the hardest part of your cycle. Hit the weights, do some HIIT, sprints, VO_2 training, and maybe do some boxing.
- Luteal phase (eleven to seventeen days): You will have higher testosterone and estrogen levels during the first five days of this phase. You will have a higher than normal pre-workout heart rate. You will also have lower

oxygen consumption, VO_2 max, and other markers for endurance than during your follicular and menstrual phases.[38]

— Training suggestions: During the first days, utilize the elevated testosterone and estrogen fluctuation to your advantage.[39] Higher estrogen levels trigger pain-masking tolerance in the brain,[40] so you may be able to lift more weight or push yourself a little further. During the first half of this phase, use the testosterone and estrogen peak to your advantage by focusing on more resistance training or hill sprints with at least a 1:3 work-to-rest ratio.

Then, in the second half of the phase, switch to lower-intense exercise and flexibility training. This is the time when you may get more exhausted and potentially have catabolic training so consider dialing things back, especially if you don't feel like you're recovering well.[41] You also may want to bump up your carb intake because not having enough carbs can elevate cortisol levels and cortisol can be catabolic as well.[42] Yes, I just gave you permission to eat more carbs! They'll help with your performance and your mood.[43]

You probably want to avoid higher-intensity cardio sessions and HIIT during this phase. If you're tracking your heart rate, understand that it is likely to be much higher than normal. This is the time to focus on strength training.

Hydrating During Your Cycle

Throughout the course of your cycle, you can have changes in hydration needs.[44] If you don't meet those needs, it will affect you on a performance and mental level. In particular, you need to increase your fluid intake during your mid-luteal phase. And not just water, but electrolytes as well. Here are some water tips during this phase and in general throughout your cycle:

- Two hours before training: Drink 16 to 18 ounces of water.
- Thirty minutes before training: Drink an electrolyte mixture with sodium.

- Working out more than one hour: Drink a sports drink or coconut water.
- Post-training: Drink 16 to 24 ounces of water for every pound lost through sweat (yes, weigh yourself before and after). You can also have foods that contain a lot of water like watermelon. Yum!

Eating During Your Cycle

Your body can change how you metabolize macronutrients throughout your cycle. You want to pay the most attention to protein and carbs.

- Protein: You will break down more protein with increased catabolism to fuel cellular processes with peak progesterone levels in the luteal phase.[45] This is the time to bump up the protein a little bit, especially if you are training at an intense level.
- Carbs: When you are fasted during the follicular phase, you can perform better over the luteal phase, although, when fueling with carbs before training, performance is matched.[46] This happens because as estrogen and progesterone peak, your body can suppress energy stores (gluconeogenesis) where your body converts non-carb sources into energy. Adding some carbs during this phase can give you that energy.

I recognize that I don't have a menstrual cycle so I'll never fully understand what it's like to go through all the phases. But I do strongly believe that the fitness industry should pay more attention to the menstrual cycle for cis women. Change always starts with one person, so even if I'm the only trainer talking to his clients about their periods, it's a start! Just remember, you are unique in every single way, from your body to how your mind works. All of that matters and impacts your health journey. Surround yourself with people who understand and respect that.

I'm so freaking grateful I got to work with Joey Thurman! He's seriously the best trainer I've ever worked with, and as an action actress, I've worked with a lot. I was so impressed with his knowledge, kindness, and full-spectrum approach. Most other trainers I worked with were so stuck in old, rigid ways of thinking and training and it never fully worked for me. This is why I'm so grateful I got to meet and work with Joey as he just gets it! He was NOT cookie cutter at all. He personalized everything to me, my body, my hormones, my cycles, my stress, my sleep, my lifestyle, and my specific goals.

And honestly, I really believe this is what everyone needs—personalized health, nutrition, workouts, etc., because we are all so unique, especially if you are a woman who is still menstruating. It meant so much that he really honored my cycles. Where most would push me harder during that time, he allowed me to rest and recover (which is what women really need during that time). I truly believe there's so much misinformation about women's health out there, and it's people like Joey, who really study and research on a regular basis (not just men's health, but also women's health) and optimize for both, that truly make a difference in people's lives and in the world.

—Rachele Brooke Smith, actress, producer, speaker

CAN YOU LOSE WEIGHT WITH ONLY EXERCISE?

Can you lose weight by focusing on exercise only and not paying attention to your diet? This is a popular question with a complicated answer. Well, the answer is yes . . . and no. Here's the thing. When people start or increase an exercise routine, they tend to use that as an excuse to reward themselves and overeat. I get it, and I'm guilty of it myself. Before I get into the science and research regarding this question, let me just remind everyone (myself included) of an important point. We aren't children anymore. We are adults, and we are in charge of our lives, our thoughts, and the consequences of our decisions. Do we really need that cookie (or two or three) as a reward for doing something that's good for us?

Shouldn't the only reward we need be the satisfaction and pride of knowing we are making better decisions for our health and our life? Sometimes easier said than done, I know, but still something to keep in mind.

That being said, can you outwork a bad diet? Maybe a little bit in the beginning. In one study, fifty-two obese cis males lost 16.5 pounds over three months with exercise only and no caloric restrictions.[47] In another study, a group of overweight individuals lost an average of 7 percent body weight over about seventeen weeks through exercise alone and no caloric restrictions.[48] These studies may seem like great evidence that you can lose weight with exercise alone, but most of the study participants were overweight, untrained, and sedentary. So yes, adding in exercise and changing nothing else resulted in weight loss. But your body is an amazing, adaptive system. At some point, you'll either need to keep increasing your exercise or clean up your diet to keep losing weight. And you can only exercise so much. In fact, it seems as if the body has a calorie burning ceiling of around 4,000 calories per day[49] (or two and a half times your resting metabolic rate).

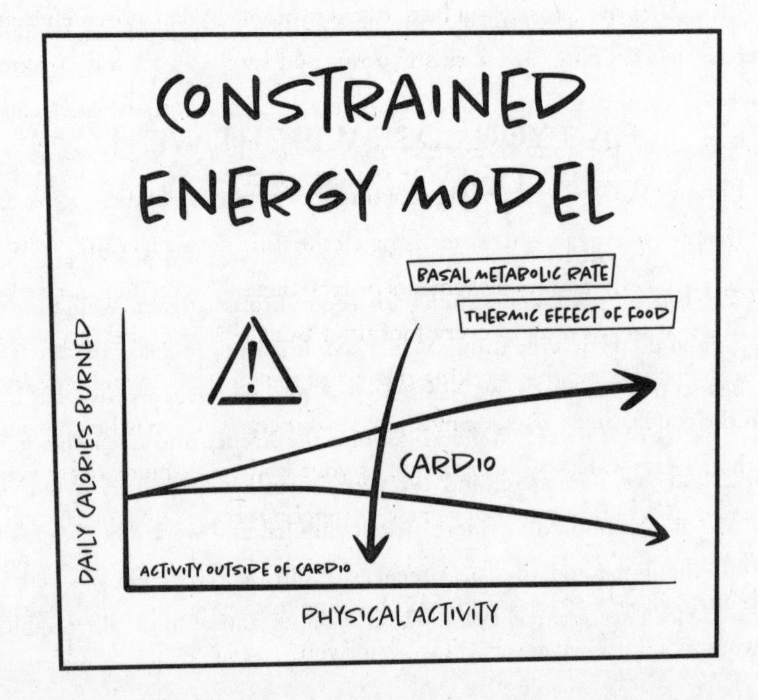

THE CONFUSING ART OF CALORIE BURN

As I've mentioned before, our bodies are smart and adaptable. They also learn to be efficient. While this is technically good, it can be frustrating as time goes on if you're trying to lose weight. Our bodies are capable of adapting to an exercise to the point where our calorie burn decreases over time while doing the same exercise.

During a 140-day transcontinental race, runners burned far fewer calories at the end of the race than at the beginning even though the exercise (running) remained constant. Extreme example, I know, but it's true even for nonathletes. One study looked at people training for a half marathon over a forty-week period.[50] Initially, the group saw about a 30 percent increase in metabolic rate, but their sleeping metabolic rates tended to decrease. As their training went on and they neared the race, their metabolic rates seemed to plateau.

You see, your body is sneakily smart. As you increase your energy expenditure, your body naturally slows itself down to preserve energy. This is usually subconscious and in the form of non-exercise activity thermogenesis calorie burn,[51] meaning the calories you burn during your everyday movements outside of exercise and sleeping. Think sitting down and standing up, walking around, reaching for things, and even fidgeting. If you think about it, the more you consciously move in the form of exercise, the less you'll move subconsciously. Not ideal, I know. That's why I'm a big proponent of being consciously active all the time. That doesn't mean you're exercising all the time. It means you're constantly aware of your body and its movements or lack thereof. Sure, you can make it a point to get your training in every morning. But then it can be all too easy to get stuck at your computer, working the rest of the day only to go home and veg out on the couch. Some days, being stuck at your computer may be unavoidable. I get that. I just want you to be aware of your body. The more aware you are, the easier it is to get in more movement throughout the day. Stand up and take a short walk every hour or so. Fidget while you're at your desk. Stand up and stretch during commercial breaks. Hit the same number of steps daily outside of your workouts. Find whatever will work for you.

ESSENTIAL EXERCISE SUPPLEMENTS

If you are looking to increase strength or performance, consider these supplements:

- Electrolytes and sodium: You have probably heard that salt is bad for you right? Well, without it we would have a host of issues, including lethargy, confusion, and less cell signaling. Taking an electrolyte mixture with 500 milligrams or more of sodium twenty minutes or so before training can actually help performance.[52] This could be as little as a ¼ teaspoon of salt or a simple electrolyte packet. Supplementing with electrolytes and sodium will help your nerve cells communicate better to help with muscle contractions and blood volume. We lose up to 900 milligrams of sodium per hour when we sweat, so replacing it is of utmost importance.
- Creatine monohydrate: Creatine is an amino acid found mostly in your body's muscles. It is one of the most studied supplements in the world and is extremely safe and beneficial. I recommend creatine to all my clients, regardless of age or gender. Supplementing with creatine helps you regenerate ATP for energy[53] as well as muscular strength,[54] so you can knock out those extra reps at the end of a set. Besides the exercise benefits, creatine has even been shown to help with mental health,[55] including cognitive processing, brain function, recovering from trauma, Alzheimer's, and depression. A typical dose is around 5 grams per day.
- Daily nitrates: These are simply foods with nitrates that circulate in the body and turn into nitric oxide (NO) when needed. Beetroot and leafy greens are the most common source of nitrates. You can get beetroot powder or juice in supplement form. Having elevated NO levels helps with aerobic endurance, power output, and muscle recovery between exercises and may help with anaerobic endurance.[56] Some vegetables with the highest amount of daily nitrates are arugula, dill, collard greens, beets, bok choy, celery, and kale.

The following supplements are great for muscles and strength:

- Caffeine: Caffeine can have a positive effect on working out if you take 400 to 600 milligrams with theanine (300 milligrams) about half an hour before a difficult workout. Taken together, theanine and caffeine have a synergistic effect and can help performance and alertness.[57] Only do this twice a week.
- Alpha GPC: Alpha GPC helps increase acetylcholine, which is a neurotransmitter that helps with muscle, memory, movement, thinking, and other aspects of brain function.[58] Taking 300 to 600 milligrams of it per day about thirty minutes before exercising can help with endurance and growth hormone secretion.
- Creatine: I talk about creatine many times throughout the book. It is one of the most studied supplements on the planet and has been proven to be safe. General doses are around 5 grams per day. (Yes, ladies, this is safe to take for you as well.) Essentially, creatine gives your body more ability to produce the ever-so-needed ATP energy to fuel your workouts.
- HMB (β-Hydroxy β-methylbutyric acid): This can help with muscle wasting (anti-catabolic) and recovery. Dosage ranges from 1 to 3 grams daily and seems to be most effective thirty to forty-five minutes before training.

Endurance can be enhanced by these supplements:

- Branch chain amino acids (BCAAs): Consume 10 to 20 grams of BCAAs before exercise, or you can opt for essential amino acids (EAAs), which have all of the BCAAs and then some. Additionally, you can take 100 to 200 milligrams of caffeine (about one cup of coffee) with an equal dose of theanine about thirty minutes before exercise.
- Beta alanine: Beta alanine has also been shown to be effective for endurance training and other performance benefits.[59] It is an amino acid and works with histidine in the body to form carnosine.

- Carnosine: This protein-building block can reduce lactic acid in the body during exercise and, in turn, help with performance.[60] Essentially, carnosine acts like a buffer to reduce the amount of acidity a muscle experiences.[61] With an increase in performance, it is thought that beta alanine can help with body composition.[62] Standard supplementation is about 5 to 6.5 grams per day taken with food, and it can last up to two hours. It can also be taken about thirty minutes before exercise.
- Citrulline malate: The amino acid citrulline malate helps with the body's energy production.[63] Taking 8 to 10 grams[64] before exercise has shown to increase blood flow, athletic performance, number of reps to fatigue, exercise recovery, and lower levels of fatigue.[65]

THE MINIMUM METHOD EXERCISE PROTOCOLS

Let's Go!

- Get at least 150 minutes of physical activity per week. You can easily achieve this in five days by taking your three 10-minute walks after each meal.
- Try to make at least 20 to 30 of those minutes some sort of vigorous activity. You can easily achieve this in five days by incorporating one 7-minute training session per day before a meal. That will equal 30 minutes of intense work with 5 minutes of cooling down.
- You can easily take it a step further by doing your 7-minute training session before each of your three meals per day and your 10-minute walk after each meal. If you do that, you will log 51 minutes of exercise per day and 357 minutes of movement a week.
- Perform The Big Three exercises followed by the Three to Be Free movements. If you can do this before a meal, it serves as a small burst of

training to get your body primed to take in energy (calories) and use it more efficiently. Try to do this at least three days a week and work your way up to most days of the week, if not all of them.

Level Up!

- Do at least half of your after-meal walks backward.
- Two days a week, do a short seven-minute burst training before you eat. This can be a quick run, brisk walk, several sets of arms, a quick leg routine, anything to challenge yourself for seven minutes. Then take some deep breaths and get ready for your meal.
- Two to three days a week, perform all body resistance training for at least thirteen minutes. Focus on major muscle groups first, then core, and then ancillary exercises.
- Do the seven-minute or Complete 180 workout once per week.
- Once a week, do a super slow rep-count full-body workout. Choose a full-body routine (ideally using machines) that consists of six exercises. You can do the workout from the super slow study earlier in this chapter or choose your own. Do each exercise at twenty seconds per rep, failing at four to six reps. Do this at least once per week.
- Once every two weeks, do five four-minute high-intensity rounds (87 percent max heart rate or higher) with four minutes of rest or active rest between sets.

Max Out!

- Weight train at least three days a week with a full-body or split routine for thirty to forty-five minutes, hitting all muscle groups for at least ten sets each week.

- Incorporate steady-state cardio (a consistent steady effort such as walking, jogging, bike riding, etc.) or moderate-intensity cardio for twenty to thirty minutes one to two times per week.
- Do a seven-minute training session two times a week.
- Do sprint training at least once a week.
- Do super slow resistance training at least once a week.
- You've mastered walking backward, and you're experimenting with sprinting backward uphill.
- Incorporate supplements into your diet.

7

STRETCHING, WARM-UP, AND RECOVERY MATTERS

Think of your entire body as a car. It needs regular maintenance, washes (hopefully), and every now and then it may need some repairs. You don't turn your car on and immediately floor it to go as fast as you can. You ease down on the gas pedal and slowly climb to your desired speed. Heck, even during races, what do drivers do before the race starts? They rev the engine. And what happens when you run out of gas? You refuel. It's the same with your body. Regular maintenance is stretching. Refueling is rest days. And easing down on the gas pedal is your warm-up. All of these are necessary to keep your body working properly and running efficiently.

Nothing irritates me more than seeing fitness influencers post on social media that you must give a 110 percent effort 24/7/365 to get the results—and the life—that you want. That is just absurd advice. You are not meant to go at that pace. As we discussed at the beginning of the book, you aren't always driving your car with your full weight on the accelerator to get from point A to point B, and life doesn't work that way either. The last time I checked, hitting cruise control will still get you to where you want to go and at a more efficient fuel rate. Think about that.

Our bodies need to rest and recover. Going at the popular social media pace, where every workout—not to mention the entire day—must be in full acceleration mode, is going to lead to injury and burnout. Even professional athletes—whose jobs are based on physical performance—take days off. Not to mention there is an entire off season. That's more like the approach we should all be taking toward our fitness. If you do not give your body time to warm up and recover, you won't be able to perform as well. In fact, it is when you are recovering from your training that your body starts to make the biggest changes on a physiological level. Taking days off is necessary for the recovery process. If you have some sort of injury, "pushing through it" might work for a little bit, but then you are likely to reinjure that area or injure another area because you are compensating. Then you will be sidelined for a lot longer than one day. Recovery is just as, if not more, important than the actual training itself.

These recovery days aren't simply lying on your ass all day long. They can be days where you focus on working in instead of working out. Working in can be meditation, yoga, a nice walk, or even some light cardio. Remember, recovery and exercise are all relative. A light run may be good for me after a leg day to help get the tissue to recover faster, whereas for someone else, that light run may be more like working out than working in so they might opt for a walk instead. The point of a recovery day is to work with your body, not against it.

By this point, you have read several methods to optimize your body and your mind. Even though you may not think so, all of those methods are going to help with your recovery. I would still say that sleep is the most important factor for your body and mind to recover. But the breathing techniques will also help your autonomic system, and, of course, food will help you recover. Even properly timed exercise can help you recover and deliver blood and nutrients to tissues that need to be repaired. So you already know a lot about what to do. But in this chapter, I'm going to give you protocols for stretching and warming up as well as more ways to directly recover from exercise and even those aches and pains from everyday life. I'm also going to give you some not so obvious recovery methods, but please don't think you must follow my advice to a T. Methods and protocols effect people differently. Sometimes just doing a little of something can be beneficial, and eventually you can hit the recommended protocol. And talking about protocols, yes—the end of the chapter has a nice straight-to-the-point list of warm-up and recovery protocols.

SITTING NOT PRETTY

We have become a society of sitting, falling, and inactivity. Too many of us sit on our asses for eight, ten, even twelve hours per day. We have gotten away from standing on our two feet, and our balance and bodies are suffering because of it. Do you know what the major cause of injury for older adults is? Falling! We get so inactive that we eventually lose our proprioception—the awareness of our body and the world around us.

Over thirty-one million people will complain of lower back pain this year, and our inactive lifestyle is a main contributing factor. It is reported that out of our sixteen waking hours, most of us are sitting for at least ten of these hours. During these ten hours of sitting, we are not using our glutes, our hips are shortened, and our posture is hunched over. When we sit all day with a forward head posture, tight hips, and glutes that provide nothing but a cushion, we are asking for problems when we stand up.

If you want to get an idea of how we are supposed to move, look at a child. Children take much better care of their bodies than we do. They are constantly sitting, standing, moving, stretching, and they have hands down the best squat form.

We are designed to move, squat, and stand up throughout the day. But instead, we sit most of the day, and that has negative implications for our bodies. Our hip flexors, for example, become tight and shortened, or overactive. When our hips are overactive they become tight leading to an excessive anterior

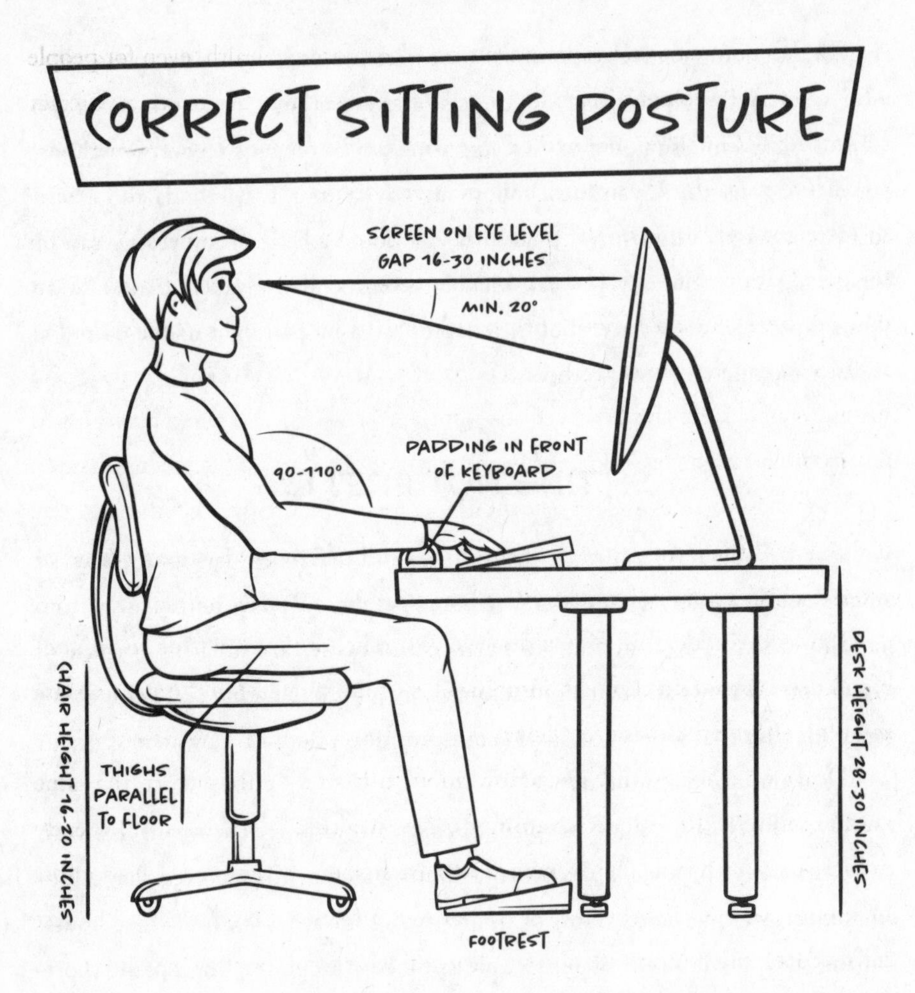

posterior tilt and excessive lordotic curve in our lower backs. This places excess pressure on our bodies and leads to injury and movement impairments.

The lack of activity also affects our glutes, which are responsible for posture, power, and a myriad of other important functions. They become inactive, lengthened, and weak. Our glutes provide us with stability, power, and hip extension. Without strong glutes, we will take excess load above or below them, hence our massive back and knee problems.

We need to release and lengthen our hip flexors and strengthen our glutes. This can be accomplished by performing simple exercises to loosen our hips and engage our glutes once or twice a day. I'll share these later in the chapter.

There's no doubt that excessive sitting is bad for our health, even for people who are active and train regularly. But can four seconds of sprints counteract the sitting? The answer looks to be yes! In a 2020 study published in *Medicine & Science in Sports & Exercise*, four men and four women were instructed to sit for eight hours a day.[1] The people in one group simply sat and could get up for personal needs, whereas the people in the other group were allowed to get up once an hour. Each hour they performed five 4-second cycling sprints at maximum capacity, totaling 160 seconds of total work. Their fat oxidation and metabolic rate were checked every two, four, and six hours after each meal. The results: high-fat glucose tolerance in the sprint group had a 31 percent reduction in plasma triglycerides and 43 percent higher fat oxidation over the sitting group! It seems as if these tiny bouts of sprints can counteract some sitting, and, better yet, the sprint group didn't perceive these sprints as being hard at all.

How do you do this? If you don't have a bike, do 4 seconds of fast squats, high knees, mountain climbers, jumping jacks, punching bags, or something else at a high effort five times every hour.

Don't want to try that one? How about this study published in the same journal in 2021.[2] Researchers examined eleven healthy individuals in their early twenties, six men and five women. Each participant performed a max effort anaerobic power cycling (PC) test three times a week for eight weeks. The test consisted of thirty bouts of all-out effort at four seconds of work with a rest time of 30 to 24 seconds in the beginning weeks and 15 seconds rest in the later weeks, equaling two minutes of cumulative exercise during the entire session, and ranging from 17 minutes total time in the beginning to less than 10 minutes in the final weeks. The results? An increase in VO_2 peak by 13.2 percent, increase in total blood volume by 7.6 percent, and increase in anaerobic power by 17.2 percent!

Even though this experiment was done on a bike, you could try the same protocol with max effort sprinting, swimming, jumping rope, doing high knees, or anything else at max effort in short bursts and still likely see similar results. As you can see, we don't need a lot of time to increase our aerobic and anaerobic power—just good intent in our efforts!

KNOW YOUR PROBLEM AREAS

Properly taking care of your body starts with understanding where you are tight and therefore prone to injury. These need to be focal areas for stretching, warm-up, and recovery. Muscles themselves are pretty dumb. If they feel like they are chronically tight and short, they will think that's normal and won't go back to where they should be. There are a number of chronically tight areas that I often see in clients and chances are, you have one or all of these thanks to our overly sedentary culture. But there's good news. Even if certain muscles are used to being tight and in a shortened position with less range of motion, you can change that with some proactive work.

- Our hips don't lie: We are in a state of chronic sitting throughout most of the day. These prolonged bouts cause our hip flexors (muscles crossing the anterior, or front, of the hip) to become short, tight, and overactive. Eventually, our bodies adapt to this position, leading to chronic tightness and pain in our backs and hips, and potential issues throughout other areas of our bodies due to overcompensation patterns. With this chronic tightness, the muscles on the opposing side of our hips,

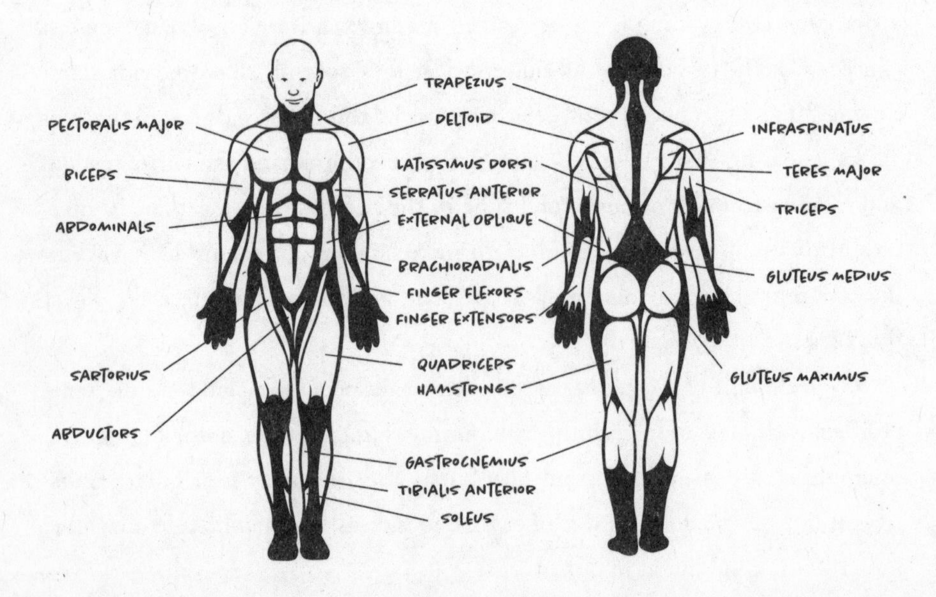

our glutes, become chronically weak because we aren't using them anymore. This is a problem because we need strong glutes for more than a great social media pic. They help power our lower extremities, walk, run, jump, and stand up. Weak glutes lead to "pancake ass." Hip flexor stretches and foam rolling (more on this later) followed by some glute exercises can help alleviate our butts being mistaken for a breakfast meal. Simply "turning on" our glutes more often can help us move more efficiently and have less pain throughout the day.

- Sit up straight: I heard those words constantly from my mother when I was growing up, and now I find myself saying the same thing to my son. Today, too many people have a condition called upper crossed syndrome. Basically, it's having a forward posture, and other names include text neck or turtle neck. Looking at your phone all day, having bad posture while sitting at work, or even how you sleep can cause chest muscles to tighten and shorten. Weak chest muscles can result in shoulder pain, decreased strength, asymmetry, and injury. Plus, it causes some of the posterior (back) muscles to lengthen, overstretch, and become underactive. Upper crossed syndrome can cause the upper back and neck muscles to be chronically tight. Consequently, the lower traps, rhomboid, and serratus anterior muscles aren't able to function properly.
- Shorter is better: Wearing high heels—or a shoe with any kind of heel—can result in chronically tight calves. Stretching out your calves at the end of the day or even throughout your day can help loosen your muscles and alleviate pain. It's also a good idea to work on strengthening your anterior tibialis muscle on the front part of your shin with some toe raises, band resistant dorsiflexion, or leaning wall raises.

STRETCHING 101

A lack of flexibility can cause a host of issues, including injury, overcompensation patterns, and lack of optimal body functioning. Tightness in one area can cause pain in another area, a condition called regional interdependence. For example, a lot of people have back pain that could be stemming from the hip flexors pulling the hamstrings into excessive tightness and a weakened stabilizing structure. Making sure we stretch and activate the appropriate areas is key to athletic performance, daily pain-free movement, and, of course, recovery.

A proper stretching program can help increase neuromuscular coordination,[3] modify blood pooling and recirculation of nutrients,[4] decrease risk of injury,[5] enhance performance, increase synovial fluid in joints, reduce muscular stiffness, recovery, posture,[6] range of motion,[7] stress relief, including headaches and back pain, and burn calories (by the way, that isn't an exhaustive list).

Our muscles are supposed to work in synergy.[8] They need to have equal functions, whether that be lengthening or shortening during a certain movement. A proper stretching protocol increases the efficiency of muscles so they can work better and get results faster without pain![9] In his book *Fitness or Fiction*, Dr. Brent Brookbush, founder of the Brookbush Institute, describes the need for muscles and joints to work in harmony to create optimal movement like this:

> Every muscle has an optimal length in which it can produce the most force. If a muscle becomes tight and short, it not only decreases its ability to produce force, but it will likely affect the relative length of all muscles crossing that joint. If all the muscles crossing that joint are no longer at their optimal length/tension, then no muscle crossing that joint will be able to work to its potential, leaving that joint unable to produce optimal force.[10]

One mistake I see people doing all the time is stretching a flexible part of the body just as much, if not more, than tighter parts. If you are trying to win a contortionist contest, then have at it. But, for example, if you already have flexible hamstrings, there's really no need to stretch them out. Instead, focus on other areas of your body that need some TLC. Overstretching an area can make you hypermobile, which could cause even more issues because it will lead to larger imbalances. The hamstring example is the most common one I see because it feels really good to stretch hamstrings, so people do it consistently but then neglect their tight hips. Further lengthening the hamstrings only make the hips pull up more, causing more anterior tilt and more back pain.

Another mistake people make is thinking that stretching should be painful. There is a big difference between discomfort and pain. When stretching, elongate the muscle to the point where you feel some mild tension or discomfort, and hold it for thirty to ninety seconds until you feel increased flexibility with a release in the tension or discomfort. You can then stretch that same area and see if you can get a little further, then repeat the process.

The Best Type of Stretching

There can be three forms of stretching if you look at it without getting into the weeds. There is static stretching, where you are holding a stretch (which could be yoga as well); dynamic stretching, where joints and muscles go through a full range of movement; and mobility, the ability of a joint to move actively through a range of motions.

Often, mobility work has a muscular component to it as well, where you may be loading a muscle in a side lunge and rotating through an active range of motion while also rotating your torso, which then increases the range of motion in your back and hips. Think of mobility as the motion and lotion for your joints to move more easily.

Overall, static stretching, where you hold a stretch for thirty to ninety seconds or more, gives you the best results.[11] Static stretching involves autogenic inhibition, where a muscle has the ability to relax and, in turn, reach a new length due to the relaxation. Doing proprioceptive neuromuscular facilitation stretching, which uses reflexes to allow muscles to relax and then stretch to their max capacity, with a fitness professional assisting you is even better. So, if you really want some help, hire a pro.

Stretching Before Training

I'm hesitant to say this because people do not stretch enough (myself included), and telling you what I'm about to tell you may lead you to not stretch at all, and that's the last thing I want. But here goes. You can stretch pretty much at any point during the day with one exception—directly before you train if you are going to lift. Why would stretching not be good before training? Think of it this way. Have you ever gotten out of bed or stood up after sitting for a long period of time and just felt like your body needed to wake up? This is essentially what happens when you stretch before lifting. Stretching lengthens and relaxes your muscles, and muscles just won't work as efficiently when they're in a relaxed state.

Studies have shown that static stretching immediately before lifting can lead to less force output of the area that was stretched.[12] Those studies were based on a static stretch for thirty seconds or more. Other studies that looked at stretching for less than thirty seconds showed no effect on peak performance,[13] but these studies were also done on high-level athletes.[14] What does this all mean to you? If you want to give a quick toe touch or stretch before your lift, you are probably okay. But don't hold it for longer than a few seconds. Instead, consider some dynamic stretching as part of your warm-up.[15]

There are a few times when stretching before training can be a good idea, and it usually involves an activation technique either on your own or with a fitness professional. These are circumstances when there is an altered length tension relationship that could hinder progress in your training or cause injury such as an altered posture. In this case, stretching the chest, for example, and turning on the back muscle will help training instead of hindering it. I provide examples on this later in the chapter as well as on my website with videos.

STRETCH IT OUT

Chances are you already know what areas of your body feel tight, but as you have learned, that doesn't necessarily mean those areas are where the problem is. I'll go over some testing protocols you can use, but if you don't have time or you are simply too lazy (had to say it) to try these tests, corresponding stretches are illustrated on my site, joey_thurman.com/minimumexercises. These include stretches for hip flexors, calves, chest, lats, piriformis, and adductors.

Tight Lats & Chest Tests

It is common to have tight lats, and people who try to do overhead presses often don't do them correctly because their lats are pulling their arms down as they try to press up, causing them to overextend and arch their lower back to get into position. There are three tests to check if you have tight lats, which are accompanied by tight pecs.

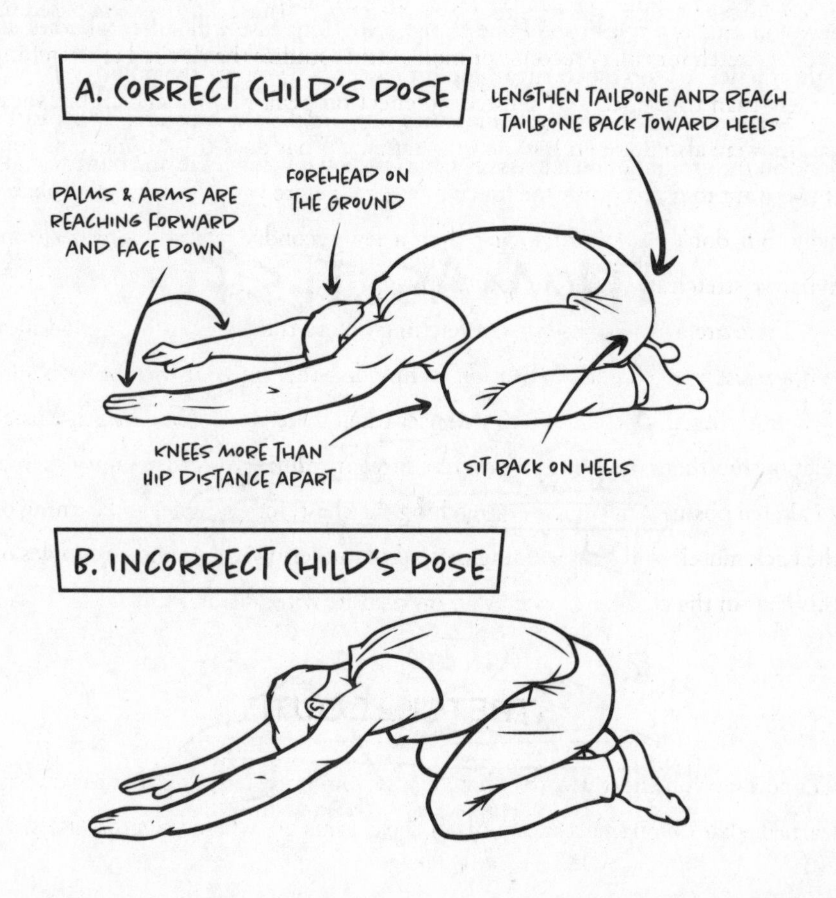

1. Stand up and reach above your head. If your hands are not directly above your shoulders, it's likely your lats and chest are tight.
2. Try keeping your hands above your head as you squat. If your arms fall forward, that's another indication your lats are tight.
3. Do the child's pose (shown on previous page). If you can't get into this position without having your arms bent and your head close to the floor, then it's likely your lats and chest are tight.

Tight Hips Test

As previously discussed, tight hip flexors can wreak havoc on your body and often are the hidden cause of back pain. Biology often determines that when we have too much or too little of one thing, something else will suffer whether it's tight hip flexors, too much sugar, too little sleep . . . you get the point.

The modified Thomas test measures how tight your hips are. This can be done on the ground or on a massage table (as shown below). Lie on your back and

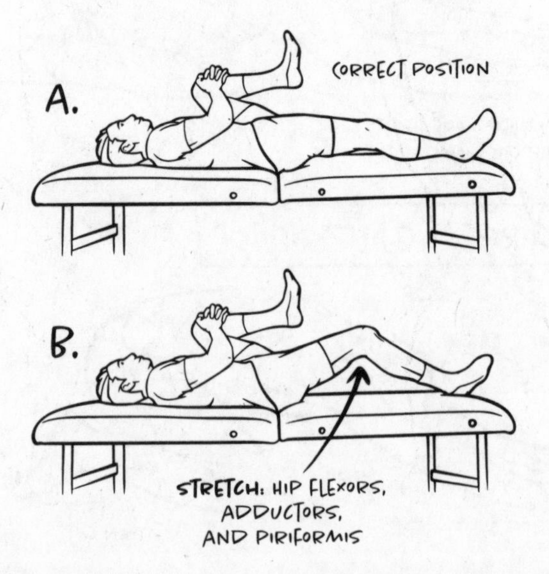

pull one of your knees toward your chest. Your lower back, sacrum, and opposing back of the leg should be relatively flat against the table. If your straight leg lifts from the table, your knee bends, or your foot turns out, then you need to stretch your hip flexors along with your piriformis and adductors.

You can also test the tightness of your hip flexors with the squat test. Start with your feet about hip width apart and your hands in the air with your biceps by your ears. Slowly lower into a squat as if you are sitting down on a chair. Don't worry if you can't go very low; just go to where you are comfortable without pain. Do ten reps without letting your heels come off the floor. When you are done, take note of where your feet and knees are. If your feet have changed positions and your heels have turned inward or outward, then you need to stretch your hip flexors along with your calves and adductors.

Now for some stretches to loosen up the areas where you failed the test. For video instructions for each stretch, go to joeythurman.com/minimumexercises.

A. CORRECT SQUAT
B. INCORRECT SQUAT
ARMS FALL FORWARD
KNEES CAVE IN
TOES TURN IN
HEELS TURN OUT

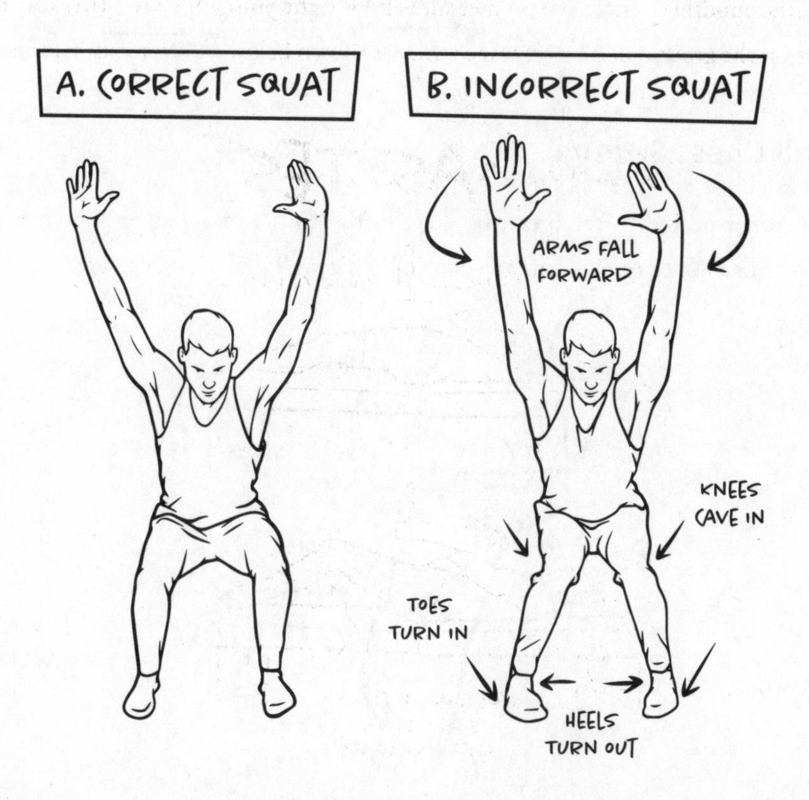

Mid-Back & Lat Stretch

Hold for at least thirty seconds or until you feel a release in tension.

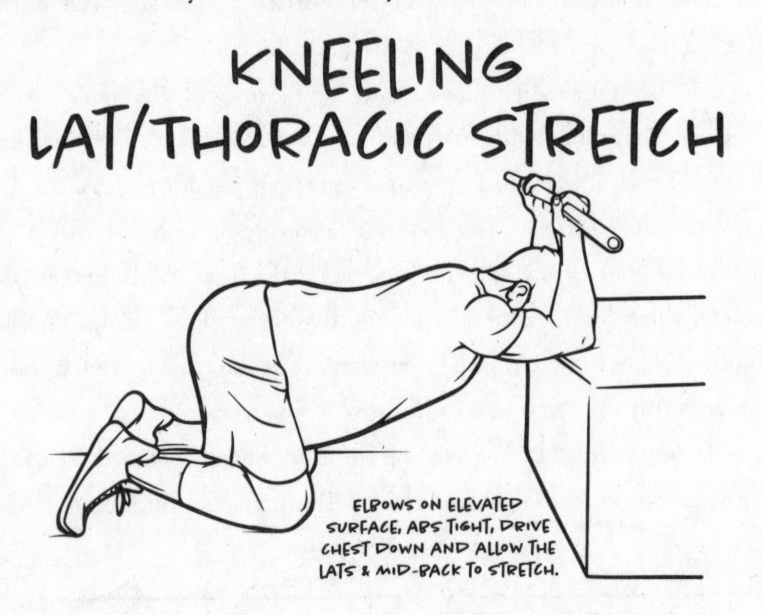

Wall Chest Stretch

The corner pectoral stretch can be done in the corner of a wall as shown with both arms at once or one arm at a time on a flat wall.

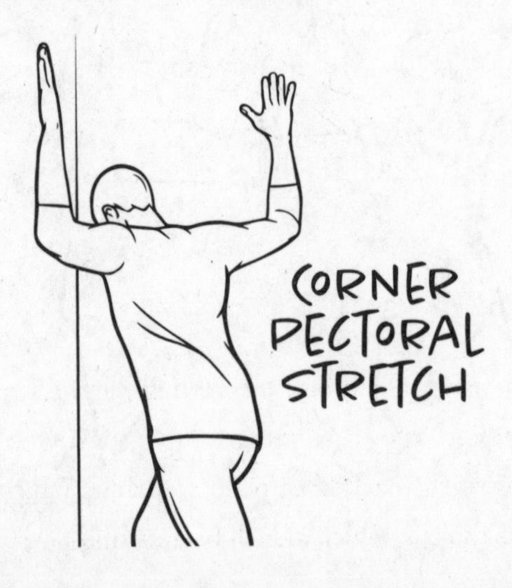

Lower Back Stretch

A lot of people complain about lower back stiffness, and I have found that one of the best mobilization exercises to get the lumbar (lower back) as well as areas of the chest, posterior deltoid (back part of shoulder), lower traps, and mid-back working well before a workout is the open book exercises. I first saw the open book setup at a seminar at the Brookbush Institute and found that ten to twenty reps of two- to three-second holds at starting and ending points can alleviate a lot of tension in some of the most common tight areas. This is great to do before a workout and any time of day. If you do not have a foam roller to rest your leg on you can use a Pilates block, towel, or maybe a small child (don't do the last one).

OPEN BOOK BEGINNING

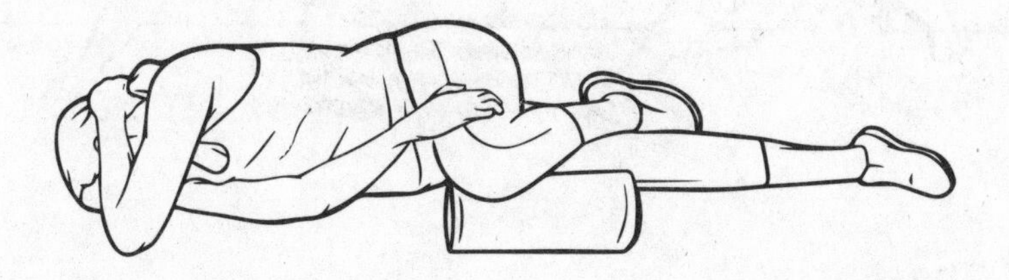

OPEN BOOK ENDING

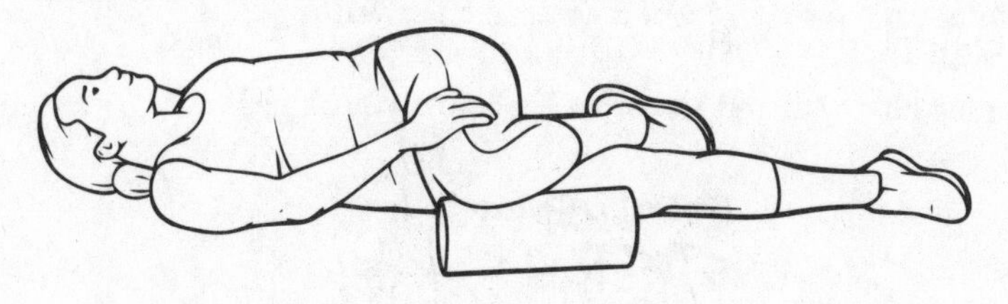

Calf Stretch

There are two variations here with one getting the thicker part of the calves that cross the knee joint, known as the gastrocnemius, with the back leg straight and the other with the back knee bent, stretching out the bottom part of the calf known as the soleus, which aids in balance and power. Use a wall or a chair to lean into this stretch and squeeze the quad and glutes when your back leg is straight and glute when the knee is bent. Hold for at least thirty seconds each. Another easy way to get these muscles is to stretch on a step.

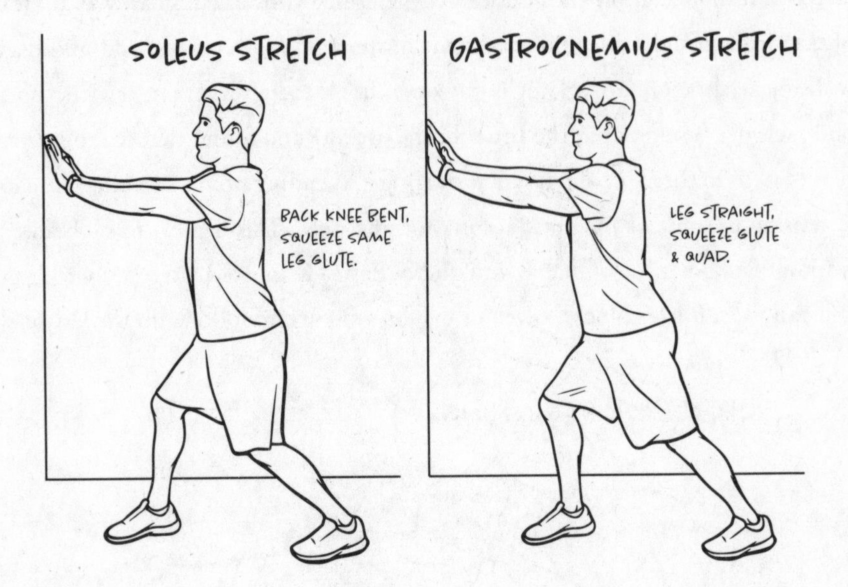

Seated Piriformis Stretch

This stretch works the gluteus medius and the deep piriformis muscle, which is often a cause of back or sciatica pain. (This can also be done on your back with the plant leg on a wall and the other leg across your knee).

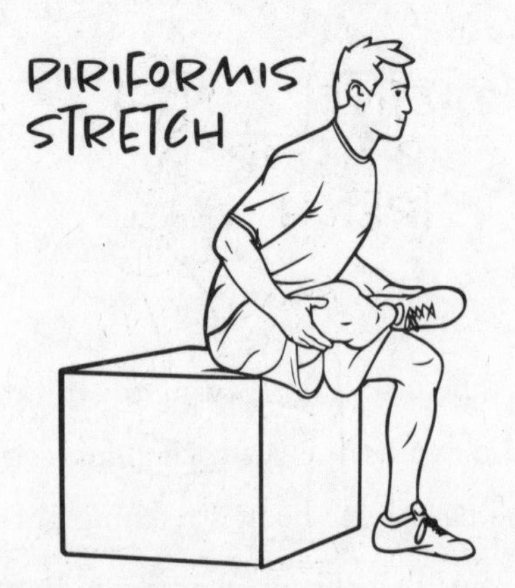

Kneeling Adductor Stretch

These muscles are prone to tightness, and you can influence a deep stretch in the anterior (front) fibers of the adductors by walking your hands farther in front of you to influence the posterior fibers as shown.

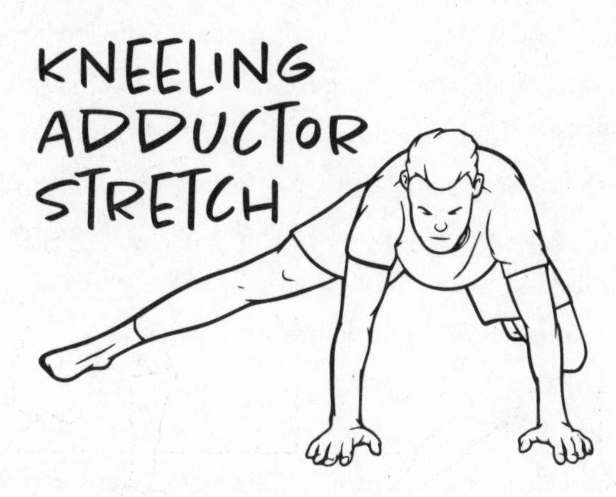

Hip Flexor

This stretch can be done with an overhead reach as shown, which will get the psoas stretched even more. Or simply do the stretch with your hands down and remember to squeeze the glute of the knee that is on the ground to go into a posterior tilt. This is called reciprocal inhibition and will immediately cause a lengthening of the hip flexor.

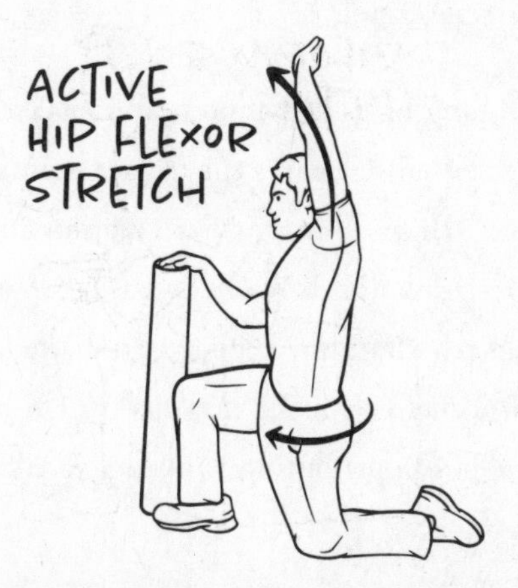

JUST ROLL WITH IT

By now I'm sure you have seen people, often with a grimacing look on their faces, using large cylinder-shaped foam rollers. But why are people inflicting so much pain on themselves? First of all, not all rolling has to be extremely painful, but often you will get that tough spot of "adhesion" in the tissue that needs to be worked out. Foam rolling is kind of like a self-administered sports massage to help with your soft tissue, including the muscle and fascia (think tissue around the muscle tissue). This has been called self-myofascial release. The National Academy of Sports Medicine calls it self-myocardial rolling. Pardon the semantics, but foam rollers essentially cause a release or the feeling of release within the tissue. But how does it work, what does it work, and should you do it?

I'll answer the last question first. Yes, you should do it! Using a foam roller is one of the best decisions you can make for your recovery as well as your performance and injury prevention. Rolling, unlike static stretching, has been linked to increased performance when used for warm-ups.[16] It improves joint range of motion pre- and post-training, and a meta-analysis showed it can help with short-term improvements without decreasing muscle performance, increase sprint performance and flexibility, and decrease the sensation of pain in the muscle.[17]

How Does Rolling Work?

Think of it this way: rolling helps decompress and relax a stiff muscle back to its natural position and essentially releases the trigger points within the tissue that are causing a restriction. This will improve circulation and prepare the body for movement. One way to think of it is if you had a dry sponge within your tissue. The rolling would help rehydrate the sponge and make it more pliable. Rolling has also been thought to help with the nervous system because it increases the parasympathetic control by contributing to overall vagal tone.[18]

The pressure from the roller is thought to trigger fascial mechanoreceptors (when triggered with pressure help tissue essentially relax),[19] which help regulate the nervous system and can be affected by the speed of the rolling to regulate heart rate and blood pressure with either slow rolling to trigger the parasympathetic nervous system or fast and deliberate rolling to trigger the sympathetic nervous system.

How hard should the roller be? It turns out that a medium roller may be the best for most people, according to a study, as a hard roller on novices will cause them to tense up.[20] When rolling, you want to sink into the roller, breathe into the adhesion, and not constrict the rest of your body, which would be counterintuitive.

What About Vibration Foam Rollers?

There are foam rollers that also have vibration technology within them.[21] From my own and clients' anecdotal evidence, vibrating rollers seem to be better tolerated. Research even points to these as being more effective over a regular foam roller, but if you already have a non-vibrating roller, there's no need to go out and spend the money on a vibrating one.

How Do You Foam Roll?

Slow your roll! You aren't trying to start a fire here. Simply roll about an inch per second, generally starting from the bottom of your body (if doing full body) and working your way up. Calves, hamstrings, illiotibial (IT) band—on the outside of your leg from the iliac crest of the pelvis to the attachment into the tibia (shin bone)—quads, and so on.

You'll want to stop on the knot! When you get to a spot where you feel like there is a large marble in the tissue, stop and hold the roller on that spot for about thirty seconds or until you feel it release. Then continue working your way up the tissue until you find another knot. When holding the roller in place, think about breathing into the tough spot with slow, deep breaths.

You can find more information and videos on foam rolling at joeythurman.com/minimumexercises.

After rolling you can either skip the stretching if you are about to train or use it as a corrective exercise protocol to move into any dysfunction you have. For example, if your chest is tight, you might roll out your pec minor, stretch it, and then do some retraction exercises to get your back muscles contracting/firing in the correct order.

When Should You Foam Roll?

Make sure to foam roll before stretching, as this serves as a primer to your stretch routine and increases range of motion.[22] If you are in a time constraint with your training, I would advise foam rolling before training and then stretching afterward. You can foam roll any time of the day, and I recommend doing it whenever you can.

One of the best ways to work foam rolling into your day, and I get this from my father-in-law, is to do it during your favorite TV show. Simply lie down, watch some TV, and roll out. Then if you can, get some stretching in. He also has my son help him, and seeing a toddler roll out a seventy-plus-year-old man is pure joy!

With all of this foam roller talk, I implore you to get a monthly or weekly massage if your budget allows.[23] Getting a massage has been shown to have a major role in psychological health.[24] People often leave a massage feeling much better and more relaxed, which increases their parasympathetic tone and recovery.

Maybe you have seen those vibrating guns in the gym and in ads—that is a percussion gun used to alleviate tension and help with recovery. But are they worth the hype and money? Yes and no. It all depends on the quality of the gun you use, how you use it, and the length of the session. In general, vibration therapy[25] has been shown to help with recovery,[26] pain, and soreness. I do love using percussion guns, especially in hard-to-reach areas.

WARMER, GETTING WARMER

I see this all too often in the gym, and for that matter with people outside getting ready for a run: they go right into training as if they were kids again. The fact is they aren't. And speaking of children, researchers looked at young soccer players and found that warming up reduced their risk of injury by 50 percent, and the severity of injury was reduced by 74 percent.[27] They also recovered faster from an injury when they had warmed up.

Warming up will not only decrease your risk of injury, but it will also help you perform better and get more out of your training, according to a large meta-analysis.[28] It may seem like a waste of time, but when you look at the numbers, you can see that warming up is well worth your time. For that matter, a proper cooldown with breathing or stretching and foam rolling shows enormous benefits as well. Stretching and cooling down after training helps increase blood flow, gets you back into a parasympathetic state, increases flexibility, and decreases neural excitability.

A proper warm-up is one that is gradual and can increase body temperature slowly, starts to mimic the exercise modality that is being performed, and doesn't tire you out for the activity itself.[29] This can be doing a dynamic warm-up that is specific to your training like light squats and walking lunges on leg days; easy push-ups, rows, and curls on arm days; and a light jog or cardio can help. You could even try a few minutes in a sauna as a passive warm-up to heat your body. This won't have the same benefits of a dynamic warm-up, but it is a quick hack to loosen up. Use your judgment based on your training. If your training is low intensity like a walk or traditional yoga, then there is less need for a warm-up. But if you're taking a HIIT class, where the instructor does not warm you up at all, make sure to do a warm-up before class.

ROLL A JOINT

When you wake up in the morning, do your joints crack and pop? And just so your mom knows, cracking your knuckles won't cause arthritis. Essentially the popping and cracking are just gases and air escaping from the joints.[30] Generally, there is no cause for concern.

When you get up in the morning, you should do some morning wake-up movements for your joints. You can do a simple ten to twenty wrist and ankle rotations in each direction, and arm and head circles in each direction. Also make sure to stretch your hands and toes, as your toes need some love, too!

HAVE HAPPY FEET

You may be wondering why happy feet are included in this chapter, but people do not take care of their feet the way they should. As a certified barefoot training specialist, yes, that's a thing, I know what I'm talking about. Here are some tips to take care of your feet:

- Stop buying popular shoes: Did you know our toes are supposed to be the widest part of our feet? Modern-day footwear has forced our feet into unnatural forms, causing bunions, pain, and less balance potential. Even back in 1905, there was an article in the *American Journal of Orthopedic Surgery* saying how bad modern-day shoes were for feet! Think about investing in some shoes, especially when you train, that have a wider toe box, instead of cramming your feet into a narrow shoe.
- Walk around the house barefoot: Think of the bottom of your feet as the palms of your hands. They are sensitive to the touch and gain better proprioception (feeling) when you use them more, even without socks on. I sometimes like to stretch and train barefoot (in my own house because that's not safe or sanitary in a gym . . . gross). Going barefoot in nature is great to do so you can gain natural energy from the earth, known as grounding. My favorite place to go barefoot is at the beach. Grounding

has been shown to help with inflammation, healing, white blood cell production, muscle soreness, insomnia, and general well-being.[31]

- Roll your feet: Tight fascia along the bottom of your feet can lead to pain and heel spurs. When you are sitting, place each foot on a golf ball and use your feet to slowly roll the balls around the soles of your feet. This is also great to do before training.
- Do toe exercises: While sitting, practice lifting your toes and spreading them out to gain more function and control.
- Play foot games: Try rolling up a towel with your feet, or even start picking up items with your toes and feet.
- Use spreaders for your toes; Before going in for foot or bunion surgery, consider getting some toe spreaders.[32] These are incredibly cheap and have been shown to alleviate foot and ankle pain. Simply put them between your toes to spread the width of your foot, and wear them when you can throughout the day.

REST DAYS ARE THE BEST DAYS

Rest days are when the real recovery happens. Questions I get over and over again are how many rest days does someone need,[33] what constitutes a rest day, and if working out too much will be a detriment? My answer to all of these questions depends on the person. For one, we all need a rest day, but this can mean a number of things. If I just started working out and doing a full-body routine, I might be sore for a few days and may need to take two to three days off to give my muscles time to repair before doing another resistance training day.[34] But that doesn't mean you can be a lazy turd. No. Your rest day can be used for foam rolling, walking, yoga, or any other form of exercise that won't debilitate you.

The common knowledge is that at least twenty-four hours is needed between training for the same muscle group, but athletes have been doing almost the opposite for years. That's because their bodies have adapted to the stimulus and can take the demand on their bodies. Plus they have recovery tools and athletic trainers making sure they are taken care of after training.

Most people who do resistance training three to four days a week should take two to three days off total, whether that is in a row or spread throughout the week. Some people who do body-part splits like arms day, legs day, etc., can take "off" while they still train, as long as they train a different muscle group. If you exercise too much, you can overtrain your body, which will lead to injury. Remember, more isn't necessarily better!

What about you weekend warriors out there? You hit it hard Friday through Sunday and don't take days off after consecutive workouts. Not to worry. I found a study looking at just this method.[35] Working out—whether it's a sport, cardio based, or recommended strength training—just two days a week on consecutive days can have some amazing benefits, including reducing the risk of all-cause mortality by 30 percent with a moderate effort of 5 to 7 METs, and even greater benefits for all of you intense warriors working at a harder effort of 8 to 10 METs! In the study, 40 percent of the participants were known to have desk jobs as well, so they weren't very physically active during the week. A minimum effort can truly go a long way . . . even if only on the weekend!

So how many days should you rest? Use your common sense. If you just started working out, you will likely need more rest. If you have been working out for years without a day off, it's time to be like an athlete and take off a season or a couple of weeks.

GETTING SWEATY WITH IT

Here is a minimum method if I ever heard of one. Get hot and sweaty without working out! I'm talking about the sauna. A twenty-year study on 2,315 Finnish men showed that those who spent four to seven times a week in a sauna had reduced risk of sudden cardiac death, fatal coronary disease, and all-cause mortality.[36] Researchers believe that this is correlated to the elevation in heart rate, which mimics low to moderate exercise, the sauna causes. And there are a lot more benefits to regular sauna use:

- Could help you live longer: Regular sauna use can reduce mortality by cardiovascular events, stroke, and even all-cause mortality.[37]
- Endurance and aerobic capacity: A study showed that regular sauna use by runners increased their time to exhaustion by 32 percent and showed an increase in plasma and red cell volume as well.[38] Using a sauna also increases heat tolerance,[39] or resiliency, which helps getting acclimated to hotter climates as well as not overheating during exercise,[40] as heat within the muscle is a main driver for exhaustion.
- Muscle growth and recovery: Saunas can help with muscle tissue breakdown as well as help protect against oxidative damage through heat shock proteins,[41] which help repair damaged proteins in our bodies and improve muscle growth post-sauna. Studies have shown[42] that regular sauna use can help insulin sensitivity,[43] maintain body mass, regulate sugar, and increase growth hormone.
- Good for the brain: Using a sauna after training helps release the ever important norepinephrine, which can help reduce cognitive decline due to migraines. Sauna use also helps BDNF, a neural growth factor, increase the formation of neurons and the power of your head computer.[44]
- Makes you pretty (yes!): Sure we all want clear skin so we can be as pretty as possible, but having healthy skin also protects us from the environment and microbes, and regulates our body temperature.[45] Saunas help clean skin by removing dead skin cells allowing the skin to breathe better. They can also make hair shiny and healthy.
- Immune boost: A study on runners showed fifteen minutes of sauna use post-run increased red and white blood cell production.[46] Additionally the same study pointed out that regular sauna use gives better cortisol control with more heat-adapted individuals.

What Kind of Sauna?

The following studies were based on traditional saunas, such as a dry sauna that gets as hot as 176 to 212 degrees Fahrenheit, not red-light saunas, which don't get as hot. But it is logical to think that red-light saunas have benefits similar to traditional saunas as they still increase body temperature. Studies have shown that the infrared, or red-light, saunas can benefit in recovery and exercise performance,[47] increase muscle mass after training,[48] decrease oxidative stress and inflammation,[49] increase collagen production,[50] and could help with testosterone production in men and progesterone production and estradiol levels in women.[51]

If you are brand new to saunas, take it one step at a time and remember to hydrate. The protocol I will give you later in this chapter is something to work up to, not a starting point! A little can still go a long way.

BRR-ING IT ON

For a long time now I have been experimenting with being in the cold. Maybe that's because I was a hockey player, or because I grew up in Wisconsin and Saint Louis and lived in Chicago for sixteen years. Brr! It's becoming evident now more than ever that we need to stress our bodies to induce a repair response known as hormesis. Hormesis is simply the body's response to a stressor that helps it better handle that stressor. For example, your body responds to lifting weights by adding extra muscle tissue, and it responds to getting cold by increasing brown and beige fat (metabolically active fat that can help you burn calories and unwanted "white" fat), which helps keep you warm.

Think about it. You probably spend most of your day at around 70 degree Fahrenheit no matter the season. You go to sleep in your house, and it's about 70 degrees (you know it should be 65 degrees from the sleep chapter). You go to your car and whether it's cold or hot out, you turn on the ac or heat to about 70 degrees. And then you get to your office, and it's, yep, about 70 degrees. We even bundle up in the winter so we don't get cold and shiver. But what if I told you that getting cold and shivering could be the key to good health and metabolism, and make you a sexy beast? Are you listening now?

Here are some benefits of getting cold (and it turns out it doesn't need to be that cold to see these benefits!):

- Getting cold after training or in general can help reduce soreness and inflammation.[52] A cold shower is fine, but don't jump in an ice bath after resistance training because it will limit the muscle growth effects of training.
- This is a fun one! It turns out that cold therapy can help increase the amount of brown adipose tissue that you have and increase your metabolic rate.[53] As mentioned, brown fat is metabolically active and keeps us warm. It acts like muscle and uses white fat (the fat that we want to burn and isn't metabolically active) for energy. Dr. Susanna Soeberg did a recent study of Scandinavian men swimming in winter.[54] After they took brief dips (thirty seconds to two minutes) in ice-cold water, they developed more brown fat than people who hadn't taken the cold plunge. And they developed higher metabolic heat production from the cold due to their body heating up. The study also found that the body became more resilient when the men varied their dips in the water with heat exposure, like going into a sauna.
- A study has shown that immersing the whole body except the head in cold water at 14 degrees Celsius (57.2 degrees Fahrenheit) increases metabolic rate by 350 percent, dopamine levels by 530 percent, and noradrenaline by 250 percent![55]
- Other benefits of getting cold are better resilience to cold weather, glucose tolerance, immune function, and higher energy expenditures.

So how do you get cold? I would like to point out that the winter swimming study looked at the minimum temperature that would induce a response, and Dr. Soeberg found it was 15 degrees Celsius (59 degrees Fahrenheit) for metabolism increases. But you don't have to jump in the cold to get these benefits. There are a number of different ways as outlined here:

- Gloves and a hat before a sweater: What? If you live in a cold state and it's winter, try going outside just for a few minutes and embrace the cold, don't bundle up but cover the necessary parts to stay safe. I go for runs in the winter without a coat and just a T-shirt on, and people look at me like I'm crazy.
- Cold showers: Just crank up the cold as much as you can take it.
- Contrast showers: Contrast showers alternate between ten seconds of warm (not hot) water and twenty seconds of cold water. Do ten rounds and finish with cold water to make sure your body gets the metabolic advantage to heat up naturally! That's a total of three minutes and twenty seconds of cold. (Feel free to work your way up.)
- Cryotherapy: Although it's a great way to get cold, cryotherapy can be expensive. Simply put, cryotherapy is a tube you get into that uses non-toxic liquid nitrogen to cool the temperatures to -150 degrees Fahrenheit and below for a few minutes.
- Rolling cold! Roll down the windows in your car in the winter without having the heat on.
- Sauna and cold: Alternate days you use a sauna with cold days.
- If you have the means, go from cold "swimming" to a sauna on the same day but make sure to finish in the heat.

HERE'S WHAT*SUP* WITH RECOVERY

I know, I know—everyone loves the supplement section! Here are supplements that will help with recovery:

- Protein: Getting protein from quality sources is incredibly important, and choosing a protein powder whether it is a whey-based powder or plant-based is essential. Get a high-quality whey isolate, and if you choose plant-based, make sure it isn't loaded with a bunch of sugar or artificial sugar. I like people choosing a protein powder that has a lot of greens and vegetables in it, which most people lack.

- Greens powder: Most people lack a sufficient amount of greens, and taking a high-quality greens powder one to two times a day can fill the void. Plus a lot greens powders have ingredients such as turmeric and ginger that have been shown to help with inflammation.
- Essential amino acids: If you are getting quality protein, you may not need essential amino acids. EAAs provide all of the branched-chain amino acids plus other essential ones you can't get from your diet.
- High-quality omega-3 or fish oil: Omega-3 is important for recovery and mental decline.
- Creatine: I've talked about this before, and the benefits of creatine can't be understated. It's one of the best supplements around.
- Citrulline malate: This helps with nitric oxide production and blood flow to get nutrients to your body and speed recovery.
- Magnesium: If you don't have enough magnesium, you will cramp. This supplement helps with muscle recovery by getting muscles to relax.
- Tart cherry juice: One study showed that seven days of drinking tart cherry juice reduces inflammation in muscles and post-exercise muscle pain.[56]
- Multivitamin: To fill any nutritional gaps you may have, taking a multivitamin is a good idea. Make sure it has a good amount of calcium and vitamin D, which help to create strong muscles and bones; as well as vitamin A, which promotes protein synthesis; and CoQ10 to reduce muscle fatigue. (You may want to supplement with CoQ10 separately as it's a powerful antioxidant for performance and fatigue.)
- Probiotics: A healthy GI is incredibly important as I outlined in chapter five.

- Bromelain and proteolytic enzymes: You might see this as pineapple extract, which is a combination of enzymes that digest protein. Bromelain reduces inflammation in the blood and body and can even be used as a decongestant.[57] Taken between meals, it can even have an immune-boosting effect by helping the production of cytokines, which are immune system proteins. There's some positive research on the effects of Bromelain fat cells.[58]
- CBD, or cannabidiol: There is good supporting evidence coming out that CBD can be used for inflammation and as a neuroprotective, and it can even help with GI damage associated with inflammation and to promote healing in traumatic skeletal injuries.[59]
- Weed: Yes, you read that right! Look, if THC is something that chills you out and you don't eat your bodyweight in protein bars (okay, maybe that's me when I'm high), then I'm all for it! Cannabis can be extremely beneficial, too, if used properly. It can help with pain, anxiety, and a lot more.[60] Obviously, use wisely.

THE MINIMUM METHOD RECOVERY PROTOCOLS

Let's Go!

- Stretch out the areas that are likely to be tight from sitting, like your chest, hip flexors, and lats. Do these stretches a few times a day. You can even do the open book exercise, which will cover a lot of the problem areas.
- Get some sauna time. Try for a ten-minute session once a week if you can. A steam shower or hot tub will work as well.
- Get cold either in a cold shower or in a cold body of water. Try to work yourself up to a total of eleven minutes per week.

Level Up!

- Before every single gym workout (or home resistance training), perform a five- to ten-minute foam-rolling session followed by some activation of areas that are tight.
- Start to incorporate some of the recovery supplements.
- Add at least one recovery day per week where you do yoga, a stretching routine, or some form of working in. This can even be a nice walk in nature (without shoes and socks, if possible).
- Work your way up to the following weekly hot/cold protocol:
  - Get cold: For more resilience and adaptiveness, get cold one time weekly for one to three minutes.
  - Metabolism: To elevate your metabolic rate, get cold two to three times weekly for a total of eleven minutes.
  - Recovery: Get cold with a cold shower for three to six minutes after training but not immediately following resistance training. Wait at least four hours, but a cold shower is okay.
  - Heat: Aim for a total of fifty-seven minutes per week of sauna exposure, whether that is in one session (not advised for beginners) or cumulative over multiple sessions.

Max Out!

- Focus your stretching on the problem areas that are tight and prioritize symmetry.
- Perform a warm-up routine before every training session.
- Perform cooldown stretching after every training session.
- Get weekly or biweekly massages, or go to a chiropractor, physical therapist, or acupuncturist.

8

THE MINIMUM METHOD

A Day in the Life

Combining everything we've learned in this book, let's walk through what a day in the life of the Minimum Method looks like for each category.

LET'S GO!

You go to bed and wake up at a consistent time every day. You're using light to your advantage by managing exposure to artificial light (including screen time) before bed and using the setting sun to help you wind down. You have a bedtime ritual that enables you to fully relax before attempting to fall asleep. Your sleep environment is cool, dark, quiet, and electronics-free.

When you wake up, you don't immediately look at your phone. Instead, you spend a couple of minutes intentionally thinking about your day, what you want to accomplish, and what you're grateful for. You have a rising ritual or stretches and breathing exercises that help you get ready for the day. You get some form of natural light first thing in the morning, whether it's on a walk or through a window. If you shower in the morning, you end it with some cold water. You don't eat right away (unless you get hangry), allowing for twelve to sixteen hours between dinner and breakfast, and your breakfast consists of whole foods. You wait at least an hour after waking up before having a cup of coffee.

You celebrate small wins. You're honest with yourself about what makes you feel good and what doesn't, and you reinforce positive feedback loops. You are aware of your level of stress and proactively deploy strategies to manage it. You actively work on changing your routines to keep your brain fresh, switching up everything from where you park to your training routine. You've learned how to breathe correctly, and consistently work on breathing through your nose. You proactively use breathwork to de-stress. If you snore, you're actively doing tongue and face exercises.

You're taking short walks after every meal, sometimes even backward. You often do short burst training before your meals. You work on strengthening your back and core daily. You've cut processed foods from your diet and primarily fuel and nourish yourself with whole foods. You eat dinner earlier, allowing your body time to digest your food before bed. You eat slower and more mindfully and fully recognize and appreciate your food. Every hour or two, you make an effort to stand up and walk around for a couple of minutes. Sometimes you even throw in some squats, push-ups, or jumping jacks to get your heart rate up.

You stretch regularly and wear compression gear when sitting for long periods of time. You're experimenting with temperatures through saunas and cold showers.

LEVEL UP!

Everything in *Let's Go!* plus this:

You proactively manage your body temperature leading up to bedtime. You make sure you go to bed hydrated and relaxed by doing light stretches or breathing exercises. You use a sleep tracker to help you better understand and optimize your sleep.

Your day is scheduled to optimize your sleep chronotype. You take a brisk ten- to fifteen-minute walk upon waking. If it's cold outside, you embrace the shiver! You do your training during the time of day dictated by your sleep chronotype. After you train, your shower incorporates some cold water, with the goal to get up to eleven minutes of cold exposure. You're experimenting with fasted training and either refuel within two hours after your workout or have some EAAs if you're extending your fast.

Every day you make it a point to move, have meaningful engagement, practice mindfulness, and try to master something new. Your diet intentionally includes foods proven to help with mental health. You're starting to develop a regular meditation practice. You use music to help you focus or relax when needed. You're aware of your breathing throughout the day and all activities, and are actively working to increase your CP. You practice Wim Hof breathing at least once a week.

You've dialed in your calories and protein intake, understanding how much fuel you need to reach your goals. All your calories come from healthy, whole food sources. You make a conscious effort not to overeat, stopping when you feel just short of being full. You practice mindful eating strategies that help you slow down and fully digest your food. If you have digestion issues, you do the Thirty-Day Belly Bounce Back to identify which foods are an issue for you.

You do regular burst workouts before you eat. Many of your after-meal walks are done backward. You're resistance training two to three days a week while also incorporating slow training. You do HIIT workouts sparingly. You prioritize your warm-up before every training session. You spend at least one day a week focused on recovery and working in vs. working out. You're taking supplements that aid in recovery and working with hot and cold temperatures to optimize it.

MAX OUT!

Everything in *Let's Go!* and *Level Up!* plus this:

You watch your nutrient intake to ensure nothing interferes with your sleep. If you have allergies, you don't bring allergens to bed with you. You have a strong meditation practice and are experimenting with listening to binaural beats before bed.

You play games with friends or family to consistently challenge your brain. You're experimenting with supplements to aid in mental clarity. You are becoming a Wim Hof breathing pro, and your CP is almost forty seconds.

You've dialed in all aspects of your cooking, including which oils you use. You strategically eat your food to mitigate blood sugar spikes. You're experimenting with the best way to get your overall calorie intake.

You have a consistent exercise routine that incorporates full-body weight training, slow resistance training, steady-state cardio, and sprints. You regularly walk backward and are practicing sprinting backward uphill. You're experimenting with supplements to help enhance your exercise routine.

You have a regular stretching routine that prioritizes symmetry. You are committed to both your warm and cooldown routines. You've brought in support to help with your recovery in the form of massages, physical therapy, or acupuncture.

Final Thoughts

Wow, you made it! Whether you read this book cover to cover or took the à la carte approach and switched from chapter to chapter, I'm happy for you. Considering you're reading this chapter, chances are you read it cover to cover. That's amazing! You have decided to make a better life for you and your loved ones. Hopefully, you have started to implement the minimum methods in this book already, or maybe you read it to start thinking about getting better. That right there is change!

GETTING BACK ON TRACK IS AS SIMPLE AS GETTING BACK ON TRACK

Remember when I told you that you were going to fail? You will, and that is okay! But I don't want you to look at missing your ten-minute walk one day as a failure. I want you to look at it as an opportunity to make it up and do better. It's an opportunity to grow and change. An opportunity to change your negative patterns and replace them with ones that enhance your health and your life.

This is why I say getting back on track is as simple as getting back on track. Don't worry about getting an extra walk or training burst in. Don't limit your food intake because you ate poorly the previous day. Don't punish yourself. Simply get back to the plan.

Remember, your minimum right now is someone else's maximum. Just getting started puts you a step ahead of much of the pack. Never lose sight of that and always be grateful for it. And know that there will come a day when you need more than the minimum, and that is amazing! I want you to be excited to push yourself more, but I never want you to push yourself too much. Stay out of the fitness myth mindsets we discussed in the beginning of the book. Part of getting the maximum is knowing your limitations.

There are always new goals to set and new heights to go after. And when you're ready for more, I'll be here to help you get there. Until then, go master the Minimum Method!

LOOK BACK ONLY TO MOVE FORWARD

Think back to before you started reading this book. What was your mindset like? What did you believe about yourself or not believe about yourself? What was the discouraging voice in your head constantly telling you?

Now, I want you to compare that to how you're feeling right now in this moment. Have you overcome some of your past limiting beliefs? Do you have any newfound beliefs in yourself and your ability to change your life? At the very least, is your mind just a little bit more open than it was before? Take an assessment of where you were and where you are now. Hopefully you see a lot of change.

I want you to be open to new things and allow your mind to be changed. The amazing thing about life is that we have the free will to change our minds and our beliefs.

I want to thank you for choosing me to help you in your life. Working on this book and this guide has changed me forever. But most importantly, I want to thank you for choosing yourself!

Now go out in the world. Be your own light. Be the shining spot for someone else.

—Joey

Acknowledgments

Wow, where do I begin? I guess to quote myself . . . the beginning.

This book was a labor of love, tears, and often frustrations; you should know by now I'm honest. I can't believe it's done.

Thank you so much to my good friend Dr. Ian Smith for pushing me to write another book.

Kevin Hauswirth for helping me come up with this concept.

Aaron Alexander for the intro to my amazing agent, Jaidree Braddix at Park & Fine.

Kacie Main Conant for helping me every single week make this book what it is today.

BenBella Books for having faith in me.

Frank Martinelli for his brilliant artwork.

My clients throughout the years for always pushing me to do more and believe in myself the way I believe in them.

My family, who has always been there along the way to support all of my crazy ideas. My in-laws, Dean and Voula Galanis, there are literally no words I can put on a page to express how much I appreciate what you do for us—you are all love! My son, Frederic, you inspire me every single day to keep on pushing for you. I hope one day you are proud to say I am your dad!

And of course my wife, Maria. I know I am not the easiest person to be married to, with my crazy schedule, ups and downs, and sometimes farfetched ideas. I just want you to know that you are appreciated, you are loved, and I will always and forever be yours!

Love to you all,

J

Notes

CHAPTER 1: YOU MUST UNLEARN TO LEARN

1. "The U.S. Weight Loss & Diet Control Market," Research and Markets, March 2021, https://www.researchandmarkets.com/reports/5313560/the-u-s-weight-loss-and-diet-control-market
2. "Adult Obesity Prevalence Maps," CDC, https://www.cdc.gov/obesity/data/prevalence-maps.html
3. "Causes of Obesity," CDC, https://www.cdc.gov/obesity/basics/causes.html
4. "Calculating Body Frame Size," MedlinePlus, updated August 13, 2020, https://medlineplus.gov/ency/imagepages/17182.htm
5. Emma Hitt, "Muscle Mass Linked to Risk for Insulin Resistance," *Medscape*, August 4, 2011, https://www.medscape.com/viewarticle/747526

CHAPTER 2: REST ASSURED, SLEEP MATTERS

1. Tianna Hicklin, "Molecular ties between lack of sleep and weight gain," *National Institutes of Health*, March 22, 2016, https://www.nih.gov/news-events/nih-research-matters/molecular-ties-between-lack-sleep-weight-gain
2. Marie-Pierre St-Onge et al., "Sleep restriction leads to increased activation of brain regions sensitive to food stimuli," *American Journal of Clinical Nutrition* 95, no. 4 (2012): 818–24, https://pubmed.ncbi.nlm.nih.gov/22357722/
3. Anja Bosy-Westphal et al., "Influence of partial sleep deprivation on energy balance and insulin sensitivity in healthy women," *Obesity Facts* 1, no. 5 (2008): 266–73, https://pubmed.ncbi.nlm.nih.gov/20054188/
4. S Yi et al., "Short sleep duration in association with CT-scanned abdominal fat areas: the Hitachi Health Study," *International Journal of Obesity* 37, no. 1 (2013): 129–34, https://pubmed.ncbi.nlm.nih.gov/22349574/

5. Se Eun Park et al., "The association between sleep duration and general and abdominal obesity in Koreans: data from the Korean National Health and Nutrition Examination Survey, 2001 and 2005," *Obesity (Silver Spring, Md.)* 17, no. 4 (2009): 767–71, https://pubmed.ncbi.nlm.nih.gov/19180067/
6. Lee Di Milia et al., "The association between short sleep and obesity after controlling for demographic, lifestyle, work and health related factors," *Sleep Medicine* 14, no. 4 (2013): 319–23, https://pubmed.ncbi.nlm.nih.gov/23419528/
7. Arlet V. Nedeltcheva et al., "Insufficient sleep undermines dietary efforts to reduce adiposity," *Annals of Internal Medicine* 153, no. 7 (2010): 435–41, https://pubmed.ncbi.nlm.nih.gov/20921542/
8. Ut Na Sio et al., "Sleep on it, but only if it is difficult: effects of sleep on problem solving," *Memory & Cognition* 41, no. 2 (2013): 159–66, https://pubmed.ncbi.nlm.nih.gov/23055117/
9. Institute of Medicine (US) Committee on Sleep Medicine and Research, Colten HR, Altevogt BM, eds, *Sleep Disorders and Sleep Deprivation: An Unmet Public Health Problem* (Washington, DC: National Academies Press, 2006), https://www.ncbi.nlm.nih.gov/books/NBK19961/
10. "Sleep Apnea," Sleep Foundation, updated March 25, 2022, https://www.sleepfoundation.org/sleep-apnea
11. Nick McKeehan, "Sleep Apnea and the Risk of Alzheimer's Disease," *Cognitive Vitality*, February 16, 2021, https://www.alzdiscovery.org/cognitive-vitality/blog/sleep-apnea-and-the-risk-of-alzheimers-disease
12. K. Spiegel et al., "Impact d'une dette de sommeil sur les rythmes physiologiques" [Impact of sleep debt on physiological rhythms], *Revue Neurologique* 159, no. 11 Suppl (2003): 6S11–20, https://pubmed.ncbi.nlm.nih.gov/14646794/
13. Jung-Kyu Choi et al., "Association between short sleep duration and high incidence of metabolic syndrome in midlife women," *Tohoku Journal of Experimental Medicine* 225, no. 3 (2011): 187–93, https://pubmed.ncbi.nlm.nih.gov/22001675/
14. Orfeu M. Buxton et al., "Sleep Restriction for 1 Week Reduces Insulin Sensitivity in Healthy Men," *Diabetes* 59, no. 9 (2010): 2126–33, https://www.ncbi.nlm.nih.gov/pmc/articles/PMC2927933/
15. Francesco P. Cappuccio et al., "Quantity and quality of sleep and incidence of type 2 diabetes: a systematic review and meta-analysis," *Diabetes Care* 33, no. 2 (2010): 414–20, https://pubmed.ncbi.nlm.nih.gov/19910503/
16. P. Zimmet et al., "The Circadian Syndrome: is the Metabolic Syndrome and much more!" *Journal of Internal Medicine* 286, no. 2 (2019): 181–91, https://onlinelibrary.wiley.com/doi/10.1111/joim.12924
17. Stoyan Dimitrov et al., "Ga$_s$-coupled receptor signaling and sleep regulate integrin activation of human antigen-specific T cells," *Journal of Experimental Medicine* 216, no. 3 (2019): 517–26, https://rupress.org/jem/article/216/3/517/120367/G-s-coupled-receptor-signaling-and-sleep-regulate

18. Alexander J. Scott et al., "Does improving sleep lead to better mental health? A protocol for a meta-analytic review of randomised controlled trials," *BMJ Open* 7, no. 9 (2017), https://bmjopen.bmj.com/content/7/9/e016873
19. Abhishek S. Prayag et al., "Melatonin suppression is exquisitely sensitive to light and primarily driven by melanopsin in humans," *Journal of Pineal Research* 66, no. 4 (2019), https://pubmed.ncbi.nlm.nih.gov/30697806/
20. Scott Gavura, "Melatonin: What's on the label isn't in the bottle," *Science-Based Medicine*, March 9, 2017, https://sciencebasedmedicine.org/melatonin-whats-on-the-label-isnt-in-the-bottle/
21. R. H. Waring, "Report on Absorption of magnesium sulfate (Epsom salts) across the skin," *Magnesium Online Library*, January 10, 2004, https://www.mgwater.com/transdermal.shtml
22. Jackson Williams et al., "L-Theanine as a Functional Food Additive: Its Role in Disease Prevention and Health Promotion," *Beverages* 2, no. 2 (2016): 13, https://www.mdpi.com/2306-5710/2/2/13/htm
23. Janmejai K. Srivastava et al., "Chamomile: A herbal medicine of the past with bright future," *Molecular Medicine Reports* 3, no. 6 (2010): 895–901, https://www.ncbi.nlm.nih.gov/pmc/articles/PMC2995283/
24. "Supplement Guides," Examine, https://examine.com/guides/#core-supplements
25. "Kava," University of Michigan Health, updated September 23, 2020, https://www.uofmhealth.org/health-library/tn7356spec
26. Azmi Mohd et al., "Cortisol on Circadian Rhythm and Its Effect on Cardiovascular System," *International Journal of Environmental Research and Public Health* 18, no. 2 (January 14, 2021): 676, https://www.ncbi.nlm.nih.gov/pmc/articles/PMC7830980/
27. Natalie D. Dautovich et al., "A systematic review of the amount and timing of light in association with objective and subjective sleep outcomes in community-dwelling adults," *Sleep Health* 5, no. 1 (2019): 31–48, https://www.ncbi.nlm.nih.gov/pmc/articles/PMC6814154/
28. Kazue Okamoto-Mizuno and Koh Mizuno, "Effects of thermal environment on sleep and circadian rhythm," *Journal of Physiological Anthropology* 31, no. 1 (2012): 14, https://pubmed.ncbi.nlm.nih.gov/22738673/
29. Paul Lee et al., "Temperature-Acclimated Brown Adipose Tissue Modulates Insulin Sensitivity in Humans," *Diabetes* 63, no. 11 (2014): 3686–98, https://diabetesjournals.org/diabetes/article/63/11/3686/34165/Temperature-Acclimated-Brown-Adipose-Tissue
30. Matthew Whittle, "The Best Sounds for Sleep," Sleep.org, updated February 11, 2022, https://www.uofmhealth.org/health-library/tn7356spec
31. Jeff Dyche et al., "Effects of power frequency electromagnetic fields on melatonin and sleep in the rat," *Emerging Health Threats Journal* 5 (2012), https://www.ncbi.nlm.nih.gov/pmc/articles/PMC3334267/

CHAPTER 3: BRAIN POWER

1. Wolfram Schultz, "Dopamine reward prediction error coding," *Dialogues in Clinical Neuroscience* 18, no. 1 (2016): 23–32, https://www.ncbi.nlm.nih.gov/pmc/articles/PMC4826767/
2. Melanie Maya Kaelberer et al., "Neuropod Cells: The Emerging Biology of Gut-Brain Sensory Transduction," *Annual Review of Neuroscience* 43 (2020): 337–353, https://www.ncbi.nlm.nih.gov/pmc/articles/PMC7573801/
3. Katrina Ray, "Neuropod cells—sensing a sweet spot in the gut," *Nature Reviews Gastroenterology & Hepatology* 19, no. 147 (2022), https://www.nature.com/articles/s41575-022-00582-1
4. Felice N. Jacka et al., "A randomised controlled trial of dietary improvement for adults with major depression (the 'SMILES' trial)," *BMC Medicine* 15, no. 23 (2017), https://bmcmedicine.biomedcentral.com/articles/10.1186/s12916-017-0791-y
5. Laura R. LaChance and Drew Ramsey, "Antidepressant foods: An evidence-based nutrient profiling system for depression," *World Journal of Psychiatry* 8, no. 3 (2018): 97–104, https://www.ncbi.nlm.nih.gov/pmc/articles/PMC6147775/
6. Janelle Weaver, "Fermented-food diet increases microbiome diversity, decreases inflammatory proteins, study finds," Stanford Medicine, July 12, 2021, https://med.stanford.edu/news/all-news/2021/07/fermented-food-diet-increases-microbiome-diversity-lowers-inflammation
7. Janina Krell-Roesch et al., "Quantity and quality of mental activities and the risk of incident mild cognitive impairment," *Neurology* 93, no. 6 (2019), https://n.neurology.org/content/93/6/e548
8. Helen Brooker et al., "An online investigation of the relationship between the frequency of word puzzle use and cognitive function in a large sample of older adults," *International Journal of Geriatric Psychiatry* 34, no. 7 (2019): 921–31, https://onlinelibrary.wiley.com/doi/abs/10.1002/gps.5033
9. Robert S. Wilson et al., "Cognitive Activity and Onset Age of Incident Alzheimer Disease Dementia," *Neurology* 97, no. 9 (2021), https://n.neurology.org/content/97/9/e922
10. "Stress relief from laughter? It's no joke," Mayo Clinic, July 29, 2021, https://www.mayoclinic.org/healthy-lifestyle/stress-management/in-depth/stress-relief/art-20044456
11. Frances H. Rauscher, Gordon L. Shaw, and Catherine N. Ky, "Music and spatial task performance," *Nature* 365 (1993): 611, https://www.nature.com/articles/365611a0
12. Christoper F. Chabris, "Prelude or requiem for the 'Mozart effect'?" *Nature* 400 (1999): 826–27, https://www.nature.com/articles/23608#B1
13. Emily Singer, "Molecular basis for Mozart effect revealed," *New Scientist*, April 23, 2004, https://www.newscientist.com/article/dn4918-molecular-basis-for-mozart-effect-revealed/

14. Sabine Hein et al., "Systematic Review of the Effects of Blueberry on Cognitive Performance as We Age," *Journals of Gerontology, Series A, Biological Sciences and Medical Sciences* 74, no. 7 (2019): 984–995, https://pubmed.ncbi.nlm.nih.gov/30941401/

CHAPTER 4: BREATHWORK IS THE BEST WORK

1. Vivek Kumar Sharma et al., "Effect of fast and slow pranayama on perceived stress and cardiovascular parameters in young health-care students," *International Journal of Yoga* 6, no. 2 (2013): 104–110, https://www.ijoy.org.in/article.asp?issn=0973-6131;year=2013;volume=6;issue=2;spage=104;epage=110;aulast=Sharma
2. "Your lungs and exercise," *Breathe* (Sheffield, England) 12, no. 1 (2016): 97–100, https://www.ncbi.nlm.nih.gov/pmc/articles/PMC4818249/
3. T. Douglas Bradley and John S. Floras, eds., *Sleep Apnea: Implications in Cardiovascular and Cerebrovascular Disease* (New York: Marcel Dekker, 2000), 272
4. Jeong-Whun Kim et al., "Relationship Between Snoring Intensity and Severity of Obstructive Sleep Apnea," *Clinical and Experimental Otorhinolaryngology* 8, no. 4 (2015): 376–80, https://www.ncbi.nlm.nih.gov/pmc/articles/PMC4661254/
5. Roshan K. Verma et al., "Oropharyngeal exercises in the treatment of obstructive sleep apnoea: our experience," *Sleep & Breathing = Schlaf & Atmung* 20, no. 4 (2016): 1193–1201, https://pubmed.ncbi.nlm.nih.gov/26993338/
6. Cláudia Maria de Felício et al., "Obstructive sleep apnea: focus on myofunctional therapy," *Nature and Science of Sleep* 10, (2018): 271–286, https://www.ncbi.nlm.nih.gov/pmc/articles/PMC6132228/
7. Kátia C. Guimarães et al., "Effects of oropharyngeal exercises on patients with moderate obstructive sleep apnea syndrome," *American Journal of Respiratory and Critical Care Medicine* 179, no. 10 (2009): 962–6, https://pubmed.ncbi.nlm.nih.gov/19234106/
8. Vanessa Ieto et al., "Effects of Oropharyngeal Exercises on Snoring: A Randomized Trial," *CHEST Journal* 148, no. 3 (2015): 683-91, https://journal.chestnet.org/article/S0012-3692(15)50646-6/fulltext

CHAPTER 5: EATING & NUTRITION

1. T. Ohkuma et al., "Association between eating rate and obesity: a systematic review and meta-analysis," *International Journal of Obesity* 39, no. 11 (2015): 1589–96, https://pubmed.ncbi.nlm.nih.gov/26100137/
2. Eric Robinson et al., "Eating attentively: a systematic review and meta-analysis of the effect of food intake memory and awareness on eating," *American Journal of Clinical Nutrition* 97, no. 4 (2013): 728–42, https://academic.oup.com/ajcn/article/97/4/728/4577025

3. Alexander Kokkinos et al., "Eating slowly increases the postprandial response of the anorexigenic gut hormones, peptide YY and glucagon-like peptide-1," *Journal of Clinical Endocrinology and Metabolism* 95, no. 1 (2010): 333–37, https://pubmed.ncbi.nlm.nih.gov/19875483/
4. Robinson et al., "Eating attentively"
5. Jerzy Sarosiek and Richard McCallum, "Method of treatment of gastroesophageal reflux disease by enhancement of salivary esophageal protection due to mastication," US5730958A, filed August 18, 1996, issued October 16, 1996, https://patents.google.com/patent/US5730958
6. Herman Pontzer et al., "Daily energy expenditure through the human life course," *Science* 373, no. 6556 (2021): 808–12, https://www.science.org/doi/10.1126/science.abe5017
7. "What to know about the Bristol Stool Form Scale," *Medical News Today*, updated August 20, 2021, https://www.medicalnewstoday.com/articles/bristol-stool-scale
8. Fred K. Tabung et al., "Association of Dietary Inflammatory Potential with Colorectal Cancer Risk in Men and Women," *JAMA Oncology* 4, no. 3 (2018): 366–73, https://jamanetwork.com/journals/jamaoncology/fullarticle/2669777
9. Sophie Schutte et al., "Diverging metabolic effects of two energy restricted diets differing in nutrient quality: a 12-week randomized controlled trial in subjects with abdominal obesity," *American Journal of Clinical Nutrition*, nqac025 (2022), https://pubmed.ncbi.nlm.nih.gov/35102369/
10. Dan Garner, interview with the author
11. Daisuke Kawakita et al., "Dietary fiber intake and head and neck cancer risk: a pooled analysis in the International Head and Neck Cancer Epidemiology consortium," *International Journal of Cancer* 141, no. 9 (2017): 1811–21, https://www.ncbi.nlm.nih.gov/pmc/articles/PMC5797849/
12. Isabelle Romieu et al., "Fiber intake modulates the association of alcohol intake with breast cancer," *International Journal of Cancer* 140, no. 2 (2017): 316–21, https://www.ncbi.nlm.nih.gov/pmc/articles/PMC6198933/
13. Mark A. Pereira et al., "Dietary fiber and risk of coronary heart disease: a pooled analysis of cohort studies," *Archives of Internal Medicine* 164, no. 4 (2004): 370–76, https://pubmed.ncbi.nlm.nih.gov/14980987/
14. Joy Son et al., "The Effect of Athletes' Probiotic Intake May Depend on Protein and Dietary Fiber Intake," *Nutrients* 12, no. 10 (2020): 2947, https://pubmed.ncbi.nlm.nih.gov/32992898/
15. James DiNicolantonio, interview with the author
16. Kevin D. Hall et al., "Ultra-Processed Diets Cause Excess Calorie Intake and Weight Gain: An Inpatient Randomized Controlled Trial of Ad Libitum Food Intake," *Cell Metabolism* 30, no. 1 (2019): 67–77, https://pubmed.ncbi.nlm.nih.gov/31105044/
17. J. C. Kolars et al., "Yogurt—an autodigesting source of lactose," *New England Journal of Medicine* 310, no. 1 (1984): 1–3, https://pubmed.ncbi.nlm.nih.gov/6417539/

18. Jeannette M. Beasley et al., "Higher biomarker-calibrated protein intake is not associated with impaired renal function in postmenopausal women," *Journal of Nutrition* 141, no. 8 (2011): 1502–07, https://pubmed.ncbi.nlm.nih.gov/21653574/
19. J. R. Poortmans and O. Dellalieux, "Do regular high protein diets have potential health risks on kidney function in athletes," *International Journal of Sport Nutrition and Exercise Metabolism* 10, no. 1 (2000): 28–38, https://pubmed.ncbi.nlm.nih.gov/10722779/
20. Stuart M. Phillips et al., "Protein 'requirements' beyond the RDA: implications for optimizing health," *Applied Physiology, Nutrition, and Metabolism = Physiologie appliquee, nutrition et metabolisme* 41, no. 5 (2016): 565–72, https://pubmed.ncbi.nlm.nih.gov/26960445/
21. Virginia A. Aparicio et al., "Effects of high-whey-protein intake and resistance training on renal, bone and metabolic parameters in rats," *British Journal of Nutrition* 105, no. 6 (2011): 836–45, https://pubmed.ncbi.nlm.nih.gov/21059282/
22. George A. Bray et al., "Effect of dietary protein content on weight gain, energy expenditure, and body composition during overeating: a randomized controlled trial," *JAMA* 307, no. 1 (2012): 47–55, https://pubmed.ncbi.nlm.nih.gov/22215165/
23. Phillips et al., "Protein 'requirements' beyond the RDA"
24. Ralf Jäger et al., "International Society of Sports Nutrition Position Stand: protein and exercise," *Journal of the International Society of Sports Nutrition* 14 (2017): 20, https://pubmed.ncbi.nlm.nih.gov/28642676/
25. Arash Bandegan et al., "Indicator Amino Acid-Derived Estimate of Dietary Protein Requirement for Male Bodybuilders on a Nontraining Day Is Several-Fold Greater than the Current Recommended Dietary Allowance," *Journal of Nutrition* 147, no. 5 (2017): 850-857, https://pubmed.ncbi.nlm.nih.gov/28179492/
26. Robert W. Morton et al., "A systematic review, meta-analysis and meta-regression of the effect of protein supplementation on resistance training-induced gains in muscle mass and strength in healthy adults," *British Journal of Sports Medicine* 52, no. 6 (2018): 376–384, https://pubmed.ncbi.nlm.nih.gov/28698222/
27. Jose Antonio et al., "A high protein diet (3.4 g/kg/d) combined with a heavy resistance training program improves body composition in healthy trained men and women—a follow-up investigation," *Journal of the International Society of Sports Nutrition* 12 (2015): 39, https://pubmed.ncbi.nlm.nih.gov/26500462/
28. Alex Leaf and Jose Antonio, "The Effects of Overfeeding on Body Composition: The Role of Macronutrient Composition—A Narrative Review," *International journal of Exercise Science* 10, no. 8 (2017): 1275–1296, https://pubmed.ncbi.nlm.nih.gov/29399253/
29. Amy J. Hector and Stuart M. Phillips, "Protein Recommendations for Weight Loss in Elite Athletes: A Focus on Body Composition and Performance," *International Journal of Sport Nutrition and Exercise Metabolism* 28, no. 2 (2018): 170–177, https://pubmed.ncbi.nlm.nih.gov/29182451/

30. Eric R. Helms et al., "A systematic review of dietary protein during caloric restriction in resistance trained lean athletes: a case for higher intakes," *International Journal of Sport Nutrition and Exercise Metabolism* 24, no. 2 (2014): 127–38, https://pubmed.ncbi.nlm.nih.gov/24092765/
31. Bill I. Campbell et al., "Intermittent Energy Restriction Attenuates the Loss of Fat Free Mass in Resistance Trained Individuals. A Randomized Controlled Trial," *Journal of Functional Morphology and Kinesiology* 5, no. 1 (2020): 19, https://www.mdpi.com/2411-5142/5/1/19
32. Beate Ott et al., "Short-Term Overfeeding with Dairy Cream Does Not Modify Gut Permeability, the Fecal Microbiota, or Glucose Metabolism in Young Healthy Men," *Journal of Nutrition* 148, no. 1 (2018): 77–85, https://pubmed.ncbi.nlm.nih.gov/29378051/
33. Katarzyna Lacka and Anna Szeliga, "Significance of selenium in thyroid physiology and pathology," *Polski merkuriusz lekarski : organ Polskiego Towarzystwa Lekarskiego* 38, no. 228 (2015): 348–53, https://pubmed.ncbi.nlm.nih.gov/26098657/
34. "Selenium," Harvard School of Public Health, https://www.hsph.harvard.edu/nutritionsource/selenium/
35. Christine D. Thomson et al., "Brazil nuts: an effective way to improve selenium status," *American Journal of Clinical Nutrition* 87, no. 2 (2008): 379–84, https://pubmed.ncbi.nlm.nih.gov/18258628/
36. "Why You Should No Longer Worry About Cholesterol in Food," Cleveland Clinic, January 15, 2021, https://health.clevelandclinic.org/why-you-should-no-longer-worry-about-cholesterol-in-food/
37. Maria Luz Fernandez, "Dietary cholesterol provided by eggs and plasma lipoproteins in healthy populations," *Current Opinion in Clinical Nutrition and Metabolic Care* 9, no. 1 (2006): 8–12, https://pubmed.ncbi.nlm.nih.gov/16340654/
38. Aneta Wojdyło et al., "Sprouts vs. Microgreens as Novel Functional Foods: Variation of Nutritional and Phytochemical Profiles and Their In Vitro Bioactive Properties," *Molecules* (Basel, Switzerland) 25, no. 20 (2020): 4648, https://www.ncbi.nlm.nih.gov/pmc/articles/PMC7587365/
39. Siddavaram Nagini, Fabrizio Palitti, and Adayapalam T. Natarajan, "Chemopreventive Potential of Chlorophyllin: A Review of the Mechanisms of Action and Molecular Targets," *Nutrition and Cancer* 67, no. 2 (2015): 203–11, https://www.tandfonline.com/doi/abs/10.1080/01635581.2015.990573
40. Kuan-Pin Su et al., "Omega-3 fatty acids in major depressive disorder: A preliminary double-blind, placebo-controlled trial," *European Neuropsychopharmacology* 13, no. 4 (2003): 267–71, https://www.sciencedirect.com/science/article/abs/pii/S0924977X03000324
41. M. Makrides et al., "Fatty acid composition of brain, retina, and erythrocytes in breast- and formula-fed infants," *American Journal of Clinical Nutrition* 60, no. 2 (1994): 189–94, https://pubmed.ncbi.nlm.nih.gov/7913291/

42. G. Paul Amminger et al., "Longer-term outcome in the prevention of psychotic disorders by the Vienna omega-3 study," *Nature Communications* 6 (2015): 7934, https://pubmed.ncbi.nlm.nih.gov/26263244/
43. Alison M. Hill et al., "Combining fish-oil supplements with regular aerobic exercise improves body composition and cardiovascular disease risk factors," *American Journal of Clinical Nutrition* 85, no. 5 (2007): 1267–74, https://pubmed.ncbi.nlm.nih.gov/17490962/

CHAPTER 6: EXERCISE

1. Gretchen Reynolds, "The Right Dose of Exercise for a Longer Life," *New York Times Well* blog, April 15, 2015, https://well.blogs.nytimes.com/2015/04/15/the-right-dose-of-exercise-for-a-longer-life/
2. Hannah Arem et al., "Leisure Time Physical Activity and Mortality: A Detailed Pooled Analysis of the Dose-Response Relationship," *JAMA Internal Medicine* 175, no. 6 (2015): 959–67, https://jamanetwork.com/journals/jamainternalmedicine/fullarticle/2212267
3. Liliana C. Baptista et al., "Back to basics with active lifestyles: exercise is more effective than metformin to reduce cardiovascular risk in older adults with type 2 diabetes," *Biology of Sport* 35, no. 4 (2018): 363–72, https://www.ncbi.nlm.nih.gov/pmc/articles/PMC6358532/
4. Daizy Pahra et al., "Impact of post-meal and one-time daily exercise in patient with type 2 diabetes mellitus: a randomized crossover study," *Diabetology & Metabolic Syndrome* 9 (2017): 64, https://www.ncbi.nlm.nih.gov/pmc/articles/PMC5580296/
5. Oliver J Perkin et al., "Exercise Snacking to Improve Muscle Function in Healthy Older Adults: A Pilot Study," *Journal of Aging Research* (2019), https://www.ncbi.nlm.nih.gov/pmc/articles/PMC6794984/
6. Kyle L. Flann et al., "Muscle damage and muscle remodeling: no pain, no gain?" *Journal of Experimental Biology* 214, pt. 4 (2011): 674–79, https://pubmed.ncbi.nlm.nih.gov/21270317/
7. Benjamin C. Y. Lee and Stuart M. McGill, "Effect of long-term isometric training on core/torso stiffness," *Journal of Strength and Conditioning Research* 29, no. 6 (2015): 1515–26, https://pubmed.ncbi.nlm.nih.gov/26010794/
8. James Steele et al., "Slow and Steady, or Hard and Fast? A Systematic Review and Meta-Analysis of Studies Comparing Body Composition Changes between Interval Training and Moderate Intensity Continuous Training," *Sports* 9, no. 11 (2021): 155, https://www.mdpi.com/2075-4663/9/11/155
9. Steven J. Fleck, "Non-linear periodization for general fitness & athletes," *Journal of Human Kinetics* 29A (2011): 41–45, https://pubmed.ncbi.nlm.nih.gov/23486658/
10. Katsuyasu Kouda and Masayuki Iki, "Beneficial effects of mild stress (hormetic effects): dietary restriction and health," *Journal of Physiological Anthropology* 29, no. 4 (2010): 127–32, https://pubmed.ncbi.nlm.nih.gov/20686325/

11. Trisha D. Scribbans et al., "The Effect of Training Intensity on VO_2 max in Young Healthy Adults: A Meta-Regression and Meta-Analysis," *International Journal of Exercise Science* 9, no. 2 (2016); 230–47, https://www.ncbi.nlm.nih.gov/pmc/articles/PMC4836566/
12. Todd A. Astorino, "Effect of High-Intensity Interval Training on Cardiovascular Function, VO_2 max, and Muscular Force," *Journal of Strength and Conditioning Research* 26, no. 1 (2012): 138–45, https://journals.lww.com/nsca-jscr/Fulltext/2012/01000/Effect_of_High_Intensity_Interval_Training_on.18.aspx
13. "Vo2 Rate of Oxygen Consumption," UC Davis Health, https://health.ucdavis.edu/sports-medicine/resources/vo2description
14. Nicholas M. Beltz et al., "Graded Exercise Testing Protocols for the Determination of VO_2 max: Historical Perspectives, Progress, and Future Considerations," *Journal of Sports Medicine* (2016), https://www.hindawi.com/journals/jsm/2016/3968393/
15. C. Danny Myrtos, "Low Back Disorders. Evidence-Based Prevention and Rehabilitation," *Journal of the Canadian Chiropractic Association* 56, no. 1 (2012): 76, https://www.ncbi.nlm.nih.gov/pmc/articles/PMC3280122/
16. "Forward Head Posture," Physiopedia, https://www.physio-pedia.com/Forward_Head_Posture
17. Nesreen Fawzy Mahmoud et al., "The Relationship Between Forward Head Posture and Neck Pain: a Systematic Review and Meta-Analysis," *Current Reviews in Musculoskeletal Medicine* 12, no. 4 (2019): 562–77, https://www.ncbi.nlm.nih.gov/pmc/articles/PMC6942109/
18. D. Juker et al., "Quantitative intramuscular myoelectric activity of lumbar portions of psoas and the abdominal wall during a wide variety of tasks," *Medicine and Science in Sports and Exercise* 30, no. 2 (1998): 301–10, https://pubmed.ncbi.nlm.nih.gov/9502361/
19. Stuart M. Mcgill, "Core Training: Evidence Translating to Better Performance and Injury Prevention," *Strength and Conditioning Journal* 32, no. 3 (2010): 33–46, https://www.researchgate.net/publication/232214614_Core_Training_Evidence_Translating_to_Better_Performance_and_Injury_Prevention
20. Kristen Boren et al., "Electromyographic analysis of gluteus medius and gluteus maximus during rehabilitation exercises," *International Journal of Sports Physical Therapy* 6, no. 3 (2011): 206–23, https://pubmed.ncbi.nlm.nih.gov/22034614/
21. Saulo Martorelli et al., "Strength Training with Repetitions to Failure does not Provide Additional Strength and Muscle Hypertrophy Gains in Young Women," *European Journal of Translational Myology* 27, no. 2 (2017): 6339, https://pubmed.ncbi.nlm.nih.gov/28713535/
22. Brad J. Schoenfeld et al., "Resistance Training Volume Enhances Muscle Hypertrophy but Not Strength in Trained Men," *Medicine and Science in Sports and Exercise* 51, no. 1 (2019): 94–103, https://www.ncbi.nlm.nih.gov/pmc/articles/PMC6303131/
23. Patroklos Androulakis-Korakakis et al., "The Minimum Effective Training Dose Required to Increase 1RM Strength in Resistance-Trained Men: A Systematic Review

and Meta-Analysis," *Sports Medicine* (Auckland, N.Z.) 50, no. 4 (2020): 751–765, https://pubmed.ncbi.nlm.nih.gov/31797219/

24. James Steele et al., "Long-term time-course of strength adaptation to minimal dose resistance training: Retrospective longitudinal growth modelling of a large cohort through training records," *SportRxiv* (2021), https://osf.io/preprints/sportrxiv/eq485/
25. Karsten Keller and Martin Engelhardt, "Strength and muscle mass loss with aging process. Age and strength loss," *Muscles, Ligaments and Tendons Journal* 3, no. 4 (2014): 346–50, https://www.ncbi.nlm.nih.gov/pmc/articles/PMC3940510/
26. Timothy J. Suchomel et al., "The Importance of Muscular Strength: Training Considerations," *Sports Med* (2018), https://doi.org/10.1007/s40279-018-0862-z
27. Rahman Rahimi et al., "Effects of very short rest periods on immunoglobulin A and cortisol responses to resistance exercise in men," *Journal of Human Sport and Exercise* 5, no. 2 (2010), https://www.researchgate.net/publication/44176304_Effects_of_very_short_rest_periods_on_immunoglobulin_A_and_cortisol_responses_to_resistance_exercise_in_men
28. Suchomel et al., "The Importance of Muscular Strength"
29. "Building Muscle: How to Get Your Body in an Anabolic State," ISSA, July 31, 2020, https://www.issaonline.com/blog/post/building-muscle-how-to-get-your-body-in-an-anabolic-state
30. Yanghui Liu et al., "Associations of Resistance Exercise with Cardiovascular Disease Morbidity and Mortality," *Medicine & Science in Sports & Exercise* 51, no. 3 (2019): 499–508, https://journals.lww.com/acsm-msse/Fulltext/2019/03000/Associations_of_Resistance_Exercise_with.14.aspx
31. Timo Rantalainen et al., "Effect of weighted vest suit worn during daily activities on running speed, jumping power, and agility in young men," *Journal of Strength and Conditioning Research* 26, no. 11 (2012): 3030–35, https://pubmed.ncbi.nlm.nih.gov/22266642/
32. Gunnar Slettaløkken and Bent R Rønnestad, "High-intensity interval training every second week maintains VO_2 max in soccer players during off-season," *Journal of Strength and Conditioning Research* 28, no. 7 (2014): 1946–51, https://pubmed.ncbi.nlm.nih.gov/24561653/
33. Javier T. Gonzalez et al., "Breakfast and exercise contingently affect postprandial metabolism and energy balance in physically active males," *British Journal of Nutrition* 110, no. 4 (2013): 721–32, https://pubmed.ncbi.nlm.nih.gov/23340006/
34. Paige Burandt et al., "ACE-SPONSORED RESEARCH: Putting Mini-trampolines to the Test," ACE, October 2016, https://www.acefitness.org/continuing-education/prosource/october-2016/6081/ace-sponsored-research-putting-mini-trampolines-to-the-test/
35. Kevin A. Murach and James R Bagley, "Skeletal Muscle Hypertrophy with Concurrent Exercise Training: Contrary Evidence for an Interference Effect," *Sports Medicine* (Auckland, N.Z.) 46, no. 8 (2016): 1029–39, https://pubmed.ncbi.nlm.nih.gov/26932769/

36. Xanne A. K. Janse de Jonge, "Effects of the menstrual cycle on exercise performance," *Sports Medicine* (Auckland, N.Z.) 33, no. 11 (2003): 833–51, https://pubmed.ncbi.nlm.nih.gov/12959622/
37. Whitney Wharton et al., "Neurobiological Underpinnings of the Estrogen—Mood Relationship," *Current Psychiatry Reviews* 8, no. 3 (2012): 247-56, https://www.ncbi.nlm.nih.gov/pmc/articles/PMC3753111/
38. A. Bandyopadhyay and R. Dalui, "Endurance capacity and cardiorespiratory responses in sedentary females during different phases of menstrual cycle," *Kathmandu University Medical Journal (KUMJ)* 10, no. 40 (2012): 25–9, https://pubmed.ncbi.nlm.nih.gov/23575048/
39. "How your hormones impact your moods, health and behavior," Hormonology, https://www.myhormonology.com/learn/female-hormone-cycle/
40. Beverly G. Reed and Bruce R. Carr, " The Normal Menstrual Cycle and the Control of Ovulation," *Endotext* (2018), https://www.ncbi.nlm.nih.gov/books/NBK279054/
41. Silvia Rocha-Rodrigues et al., "Bidirectional Interactions between the Menstrual Cycle, Exercise Training, and Macronutrient Intake in Women: A Review," *Nutrients* 13, no. 2 (2021): 438, https://www.mdpi.com/2072-6643/13/2/438
42. Habib Yaribeygi et al., "The impact of stress on body function: A review," *EXCLI journal* 16 (2017): 1057–1072, https://www.ncbi.nlm.nih.gov/pmc/articles/PMC5579396/
43. Hoda Soltani et al., "Increasing Dietary Carbohydrate as Part of a Healthy Whole Food Diet Intervention Dampens Eight Week Changes in Salivary Cortisol and Cortisol Responsiveness," *Nutrients* 11, no. 11 (2019): 2563, https://www.ncbi.nlm.nih.gov/pmc/articles/PMC6893582/
44. Janse de Jonge, "Effects of the menstrual cycle on exercise performance"
45. Janse de Jonge, "Effects of the menstrual cycle on exercise performance"
46. S. E. Campbell et al., "Glucose kinetics and exercise performance during phases of the menstrual cycle: effect of glucose ingestion," *American Journal of Physiology—Endocrinology and Metabolism* 281, no. 4 (2001): E817–25, https://pubmed.ncbi.nlm.nih.gov/11551860/
47. R. Ross et al., "Reduction in obesity and related comorbid conditions after diet-induced weight loss or exercise-induced weight loss in men. A randomized, controlled trial," *Annals of Internal Medicine* 133, no. 2 (2000): 92–103, https://pubmed.ncbi.nlm.nih.gov/10896648/
48. Edward P. Weiss et al., "Effects of Weight Loss on Lean Mass, Strength, Bone, and Aerobic Capacity," *Medicine and Science in Sports and Exercise* 49, no. 1 (2017): 206–217, https://pubmed.ncbi.nlm.nih.gov/27580151/
49. Herman Pontzer et al., "Constrained Total Energy Expenditure and Metabolic Adaptation to Physical Activity in Adult Humans," *Current Biology* 26, no. 3 (2016): 410–17, https://www.cell.com/fulltext/S0960-9822(15)01577-8
50. K. R. Westerterp et al., "Long-term effect of physical activity on energy balance and body composition," *British Journal of Nutrition* 68, no. 1 (1992): 21–30, https://pubmed.ncbi.nlm.nih.gov/1390606/

51. Rodrigo Fernández-Verdejo et al., "Deciphering the constrained total energy expenditure model in humans by associating accelerometer-measured physical activity from wrist and hip," *Scientific Reports* 11 (2021), https://www.nature.com/articles/s41598-021-91750-x
52. David Ayotte Jr. and Michael P. Corcoran, "Individualized hydration plans improve performance outcomes for collegiate athletes engaging in in-season training," *Journal of the International Society of Sports Nutrition* 15, no. 27 (2018), https://jissn.biomedcentral.com/articles/10.1186/s12970-018-0230-2
53. Farnaz Farshidfar et al., "Creatine Supplementation and Skeletal Muscle Metabolism for Building Muscle Mass-Review of the Potential Mechanisms of Action," *Current Protein & Peptide Science* 18, no. 12 (2017): 1273–87, https://pubmed.ncbi.nlm.nih.gov/28595527/
54. J. Chami and D. G. Candow, "Effect of Creatine Supplementation Dosing Strategies on Aging Muscle Performance," *Journal of Nutrition, Health & Aging* 23, no. 3 (2019): 281–285, https://pubmed.ncbi.nlm.nih.gov/30820517/
55. Hamilton Roschel et al., "Creatine Supplementation and Brain Health," *Nutrients* 13, no. 2 (2021): 586, https://www.ncbi.nlm.nih.gov/pmc/articles/PMC7916590/
56. Jon O. Lundberg et al., "Roles of dietary inorganic nitrate in cardiovascular health and disease," *Cardiovascular Research* 89, no. 3 (2011): 525–32, https://pubmed.ncbi.nlm.nih.gov/20937740/
57. T. Giesbrecht et al., "The combination of L-theanine and caffeine improves cognitive performance and increases subjective alertness," *Nutritional Neuroscience* 13, no. 6 (2010): 283–90, https://pubmed.ncbi.nlm.nih.gov/21040626/
58. Adam G. Parker et al., "The effects of alpha-glycerylphosphorylcholine, caffeine or placebo on markers of mood, cognitive function, power, speed, and agility," *Journal of the International Society of Sports Nutrition* 12 (2015): 41, https://jissn.biomedcentral.com/articles/10.1186/1550-2783-12-S1-P41
59. Guilherme Giannini Artioli et al., "Role of beta-alanine supplementation on muscle carnosine and exercise performance," *Medicine and Science in Sports and Exercise* 42, no. 6 (2010): 1162–73, https://pubmed.ncbi.nlm.nih.gov/20479615/
60. Wim Derave et al., "beta-Alanine supplementation augments muscle carnosine content and attenuates fatigue during repeated isokinetic contraction bouts in trained sprinters," *Journal of Applied Physiology* 103, no. 5 (2007): 1736–43, https://pubmed.ncbi.nlm.nih.gov/17690198/
61. R. M. Hobson et al., "Effects of β-alanine supplementation on exercise performance: a meta-analysis," *Amino Acids* 43, no. 1 (2012): 25–37, https://www.ncbi.nlm.nih.gov/pmc/articles/PMC3374095/
62. Abbie E. Smith et al., "Effects of beta-alanine supplementation and high-intensity interval training on endurance performance and body composition in men; a double-blind trial," *Journal of the International Society of Sports Nutrition* 6 (2009): 5, https://pubmed.ncbi.nlm.nih.gov/19210788/
63. Benjamin Wax et al., "Effects of supplemental citrulline malate ingestion during repeated bouts of lower-body exercise in advanced weightlifters," *Journal of Strength*

and Conditioning Research 29, no. 3 (2015): 786–92, https://pubmed.ncbi.nlm.nih.gov/25226311/

64. Takashi Suzuki et al., "Oral L-citrulline supplementation enhances cycling time trial performance in healthy trained men: Double-blind randomized placebo-controlled 2-way crossover study," *Journal of the International Society of Sports Nutrition* 13 (2016): 6, https://pubmed.ncbi.nlm.nih.gov/26900386/
65. Benjamin Wax et al., "Effects of Supplemental Citrulline-Malate Ingestion on Blood Lactate, Cardiovascular Dynamics, and Resistance Exercise Performance in Trained Males," *Journal of Dietary Supplements* 13, no. 3 (2016): 269–82, https://pubmed.ncbi.nlm.nih.gov/25674699/

CHAPTER 7: STRETCHING, WARM-UP, AND RECOVERY MATTERS

1. Anthony S. Wolfe et al., "Hourly 4-s Sprints Prevent Impairment of Postprandial Fat Metabolism from Inactivity," *Medicine and Science in Sports and Exercise* 52, no. 10 (2020): 2262–69, https://pubmed.ncbi.nlm.nih.gov/32936598/
2. Remzi Satiroglu et al., "Four-Second Power Cycling Training Increases Maximal Anaerobic Power, Peak Oxygen Consumption, and Total Blood Volume," *Medicine & Science in Sports & Exercise* 53, no. 12 (2021): 2536–42, https://journals.lww.com/acsm-msse/Citation/2021/12000/Four_Second_Power_Cycling_Training_Increases.9.aspx
3. Jules Opplert and Nicolas Babault, "Acute Effects of Dynamic Stretching on Muscle Flexibility and Performance: An Analysis of the Current Literature," *Sports Medicine* (Auckland, N.Z.) 48, no. 2 (2018): 299–325, https://pubmed.ncbi.nlm.nih.gov/29063454/
4. Kazuki Hotta et al., "Stretching exercises enhance vascular endothelial function and improve peripheral circulation in patients with acute myocardial infarction," *International Heart Journal* 54, no. 2 (2013): 59–63, https://pubmed.ncbi.nlm.nih.gov/23676363/
5. Phil Page, "Current concepts in muscle stretching for exercise and rehabilitation," *International Journal of Sports Physical Therapy* 7, no. 1 (2012): 109–19, https://www.ncbi.nlm.nih.gov/pmc/articles/PMC3273886/
6. DeokJu Kim et al., "Effect of an exercise program for posture correction on musculoskeletal pain," *Journal of Physical Therapy Science* 27, no. 6 (2015): 1791–94, https://www.ncbi.nlm.nih.gov/pmc/articles/PMC4499985/
7. David G. Behm et al., "Acute effects of muscle stretching on physical performance, range of motion, and injury incidence in healthy active individuals: a systematic review," *Applied Physiology, Nutrition, and Metabolism* 41, no. 1 (2016): 1–11, https://pubmed.ncbi.nlm.nih.gov/26642915/
8. J. Antonio and W. J. Gonyea, "Progressive stretch overload of skeletal muscle results in hypertrophy before hyperplasia," *Journal of Applied Psychology* 75, no. 3 (1993): 1263–71, https://journals.physiology.org/doi/abs/10.1152/jappl.1993.75.3.1263

9. Ian Shrier, "Does stretching improve performance? A systematic and critical review of the literature," *Clinical Journal of Sport Medicine: Official Journal of the Canadian Academy of Sport Medicine* 14, no. 5 (2004): 267–73, https://pubmed.ncbi.nlm.nih.gov/15377965/
10. Brent Brookbush, *Fitness or Fiction* (2011), 149
11. Jeffrey C. Gergley, "Acute effect of passive static stretching on lower-body strength in moderately trained men," *Journal of Strength and Conditioning Research* 27, no. 4 (2013): 973–77, https://pubmed.ncbi.nlm.nih.gov/22692125/
12. L. Simic et al., "Does pre-exercise static stretching inhibit maximal muscular performance? A meta-analytical review," *Scandinavian Journal of Medicine & Science in Sports* 23, no. 2 (2013): 131–48, https://pubmed.ncbi.nlm.nih.gov/22316148/
13. Anthony D. Kay and Anthony J. Blazevich, "Effect of acute static stretch on maximal muscle performance: a systematic review," *Medicine and Science in Sports and Exercise* 44, no. 1 (2012): 154–64, https://pubmed.ncbi.nlm.nih.gov/21659901/
14. Barry Beedle et al., "Pretesting static and dynamic stretching does not affect maximal strength," *Journal of Strength and Conditioning Research* 22, no. 6 (2008): 1838–43, https://pubmed.ncbi.nlm.nih.gov/18841081/
15. Page, "Current concepts in muscle stretching for exercise and rehabilitation"
16. Scott W. Cheatham et al., "The Effects of Self-Myofascial Release Using a Foam Roll or Roller Massager on Joint Range of Motion, Muscle Recovery, and Performance: A Systematic Review," *International Journal of Sports Physical Therapy* 10, no. 6 (2015): 827–38, https://europepmc.org/article/med/26618062
17. Thimo Wiewelhove et al., "A Meta-Analysis of the Effects of Foam Rolling on Performance and Recovery," *Frontiers in Physiology* 10 (2019), doi: 10.3389/fphys.2019.00376
18. "The Optimum Performance Training® Model," NASM, https://www.nasm.org/certified-personal-trainer/the-opt-model
19. Robert Schleip, "Fascial plasticity—a new neurobiological explanation: Part 1," *Journal of Bodywork and Movement Therapies* 7, no. 1 (2003): 11–19, https://www.sciencedirect.com/science/article/abs/pii/S1360859202000670
20. Scott W. Cheatham and Kyle R. Stull, "Comparison of Three Different Density Type Foam Rollers on Knee Range of Motion and Pressure Pain Threshold: A Randomized Controlled Trial," *International Journal of Sports Physical Therapy* 13, no. 3 (2018): 474–82, https://www.ncbi.nlm.nih.gov/pmc/articles/PMC6044602/
21. Andreas Konrad, Markus Tilp, and Masatoshi Nakamura, "A Comparison of the Effects of Foam Rolling and Stretching on Physical Performance. A Systematic Review and Meta-Analysis," *Frontiers in Physiology* (2021), https://www.frontiersin.org/articles/10.3389/fphys.2021.720531/full
22. Andreas Konrad et al., "The Accumulated Effects of Foam Rolling Combined with Stretching on Range of Motion and Physical Performance: A Systematic Review and Meta-Analysis," *Journal of Sports Science and Medicine* 20 (2021), 535–45, https://www.jssm.org/jssm-20-535.xml%3EFulltext

23. Robert Standley et al., "Massage's Effect on Injury, Recovery, and Performance: A Review of Techniques and Treatment Parameters," *Strength and Conditioning Journal* 32, no. 2 (2010): 64–67, https://journals.lww.com/nsca-scj/fulltext/2010/04000/massage_s_effect_on_injury,_recovery,_and.7.aspx
24. Holly Louisa Davis, Samer Alabed, and Timothy James Ainsley Chico, "Effect of sports massage on performance and recovery: a systematic review and meta-analysis," *BMJ Open Sport & Exercise Medicine* 6, no. 1 (2020): e000614, https://bmjopensem.bmj.com/content/6/1/e000614
25. Ana Maria de Benito et al., "Effect of vibration vs non-vibration foam rolling techniques on flexibility, dynamic balance and perceived joint stability after fatigue," *PeerJ* 7 (2019): e8000, https://peerj.com/articles/8000/
26. Joel T. Fuller et al., "Vibration Therapy Is No More Effective Than the Standard Practice of Massage and Stretching for Promoting Recovery from Muscle Damage After Eccentric Exercise," *Clinical Journal of Sport Medicine* 25, no. 4 (2015): 332–37, https://journals.lww.com/cjsportsmed/Abstract/2015/07000/Vibration_Therapy_Is_No_More_Effective_Than_the.4.aspx
27. Roland Rössler et al., "A Multinational Cluster Randomised Controlled Trial to Assess the Efficacy of '11+ Kids': A Warm-Up Programme to Prevent Injuries in Children's Football," *Sports Medicine* 48 (2018): 1493–1504, https://link.springer.com/article/10.1007/s40279-017-0834-8
28. Andrea J. Fradkin et al., "Effects of warming-up on physical performance: a systematic review with meta-analysis," *Journal of Strength and Conditioning Research* 24, no. 1 (2010): 140–48, https://pubmed.ncbi.nlm.nih.gov/19996770/
29. Owen Walker, "Post-Exercise Stretching," *Science for Sport*, February 24, 2016, https://www.scienceforsport.com/post-exercise-stretching/
30. V. Chandran Suja and A. I. Barakat, "A Mathematical Model for the Sounds Produced by Knuckle Cracking," *Scientific Reports* 8, no. 4600 (2018), https://www.nature.com/articles/s41598-018-22664-4
31. James L. Oschman et al., "The effects of grounding (earthing) on inflammation, the immune response, wound healing, and prevention and treatment of chronic inflammatory and autoimmune diseases," *Journal of Inflammation Research* 8 (2015): 83–96, https://www.ncbi.nlm.nih.gov/pmc/articles/PMC4378297/
32. Sahar Ahmed Abdalbary, "Foot Mobilization and Exercise Program Combined with Toe Separator Improves Outcomes in Women with Moderate Hallux Valgus at 1-Year Follow-up A Randomized Clinical Trial," *Journal of the American Podiatric Medical Association* 108, no. 6 (2018): 478–486, https://pubmed.ncbi.nlm.nih.gov/29683337/
33. Armistead Legge, "The Definitive (And Practical) Guide to Muscle Protein Synthesis," *Legion Athletics*, https://legionathletics.com/muscle-protein-synthesis/
34. Yifan Yang et al., "Effects of Consecutive Versus Non-consecutive Days of Resistance Training on Strength, Body Composition, and Red Blood Cells," *Frontiers in Physiology* 9 (2018): 725, https://www.ncbi.nlm.nih.gov/pmc/articles/PMC6015912/

35. Gary O'Donovan, Olga L. Sarmiento, and Mark Hamer, "The Rise of the 'Weekend Warrior,'" *Journal of Orthopaedic & Sports Physical Therapy* 48, no. 8 (2018): 604–06, https://www.jospt.org/doi/10.2519/jospt.2018.0611
36. Tanjaniina Laukkanen et al., "Association Between Sauna Bathing and Fatal Cardiovascular and All-Cause Mortality Events," *JAMA Intern Med* 175, no. 4 (2015): 542–48, https://jamanetwork.com/journals/jamainternalmedicine/fullarticle/2130724
37. Tanjaniina Laukkanen et al., "Sauna bathing is associated with reduced cardiovascular mortality and improves risk prediction in men and women: a prospective cohort study," *BMC Medicine* 16, no. 219 (2018), https://bmcmedicine.biomedcentral.com/articles/10.1186/s12916-018-1198-0
38. Guy S. M. Scoon et al., "Effect of post-exercise sauna bathing on the endurance performance of competitive male runners," *Journal of Science and Medicine in Sport* 10, no. 4 (2007): 259–62, https://pubmed.ncbi.nlm.nih.gov/16877041/
39. Ricardo J. S. Costa et al., "Heat acclimation responses of an ultra-endurance running group preparing for hot desert-based competition," *European Journal of Sport Science* 14, suppl 1 (2014): S131–41, https://pubmed.ncbi.nlm.nih.gov/24444197/
40. Cell Press, "Winter-swimming Scandinavian men can teach us how the body adapts to extreme heat and cold," *ScienceDaily*, October 11, 2021, https://www.sciencedaily.com/releases/2021/10/211011110818.htm
41. J. T. Selsby et al., "Intermittent hyperthermia enhances skeletal muscle regrowth and attenuates oxidative damage following reloading," *Journal of Applied Physiology* 102, no. 4 (2007): 1702–07, https://pubmed.ncbi.nlm.nih.gov/17110516/
42. K. Kukkonen-Harjula and K. Kauppinen, "How the sauna affects the endocrine system," *Annals of Clinical Research* 20, no. 4 (1988): 262–66, https://pubmed.ncbi.nlm.nih.gov/3218898/
43. Satoshi Kokura et al., "Whole body hyperthermia improves obesity-induced insulin resistance in diabetic mice," *International Journal of Hyperthermia: The Official Journal of European Society for Hyperthermic Oncology, North American Hyperthermia Group* 23, no. 3 (2007): 259–65, https://pubmed.ncbi.nlm.nih.gov/17523018/
44. Maaike Goekint et al., "Influence of citalopram and environmental temperature on exercise-induced changes in BDNF," *Neuroscience Letters* 494, no. 2 (2011): 150–54, https://pubmed.ncbi.nlm.nih.gov/21385602/
45. D. Kowatzki et al., "Effect of regular sauna on epidermal barrier function and stratum corneum water-holding capacity in vivo in humans: a controlled study," *Dermatology* (Basel, Switzerland) 217, no. 2 (2008): 173–80, https://pubmed.ncbi.nlm.nih.gov/18525205/
46. Wanda Pilch et al., "Effect of a single Finnish sauna session on white blood cell profile and cortisol levels in athletes and non-athletes," *Journal of Human Kinetics* 39 (2013): 127–35, https://www.ncbi.nlm.nih.gov/pmc/articles/PMC3916915/
47. "SoloCarbon Infrared and Human Body Absorption FIR Assn.," https://assets-us-01.kc-usercontent.com/9832d3f0-685b-0021-9fc3-0a88ee8dfc7a/6f1de2a9-1a37-4039-937f-5464b7b004d9/SoloCarbon Infrared and Human Body Absorption FIR Assn.pdf

48. Cleber Ferraresi et al., "Photobiomodulation in human muscle tissue: an advantage in sports performance?" *Journal of Biophotonics* 9, no. 11-12 (2016): 1273–99, https://pubmed.ncbi.nlm.nih.gov/27874264/
49. Ferraresi et al., "Photobiomodulation in human muscle tissue"
50. Alexander Wunsch and Karsten Matuschka, "A controlled trial to determine the efficacy of red and near-infrared light treatment in patient satisfaction, reduction of fine lines, wrinkles, skin roughness, and intradermal collagen density increase," *Photomedicine and Laser Surgery* 32, no. 2 (2014): 93–100, https://www.ncbi.nlm.nih.gov/pmc/articles/PMC3926176/
51. "The Promising Synergy Between the Ketogenic Diet and Red Light Therapy," Joovv, updated May 13, 2022, https://joovv.com/blogs/joovv-blog/the-ketogenic-diet-and-red-light-therapy
52. Simon S. Yeung et al., "Effects of Cold Water Immersion on Muscle Oxygenation During Repeated Bouts of Fatiguing Exercise: A Randomized Controlled Study," *Medicine* 95, no. 1 (2016): e2455, https://www.ncbi.nlm.nih.gov/pmc/articles/PMC4706272/
53. Maarten J. Vosselman et al., "Frequent Extreme Cold Exposure and Brown Fat and Cold-Induced Thermogenesis: A Study in a Monozygotic Twin," *PloS one* 9, no. 7 (2014): e101653, https://journals.plos.org/plosone/article?id=10.1371/journal.pone.0101653
54. Cell Press, "Winter-swimming Scandinavian men"
55. P. Srámek et al., "Human physiological responses to immersion into water of different temperatures," *European journal of Applied Physiology* 81, no. 5 (2000): 436–42, https://pubmed.ncbi.nlm.nih.gov/10751106/
56. Kerry S. Kuehl et al., "Efficacy of tart cherry juice in reducing muscle pain during running: a randomized controlled trial," *Journal of the International Society of Sports Nutrition* 7 (2010), https://www.ncbi.nlm.nih.gov/pmc/articles/PMC2874510/
57. Vidhya Rathnavelu et al., "Potential role of bromelain in clinical and therapeutic applications," *Biomedical Reports* 5, no. 3 (2016): 283–88, https://www.ncbi.nlm.nih.gov/pmc/articles/PMC4998156/
58. Sandeep Dave et al., "Inhibition of adipogenesis and induction of apoptosis and lipolysis by stem bromelain in 3T3-L1 adipocytes," *PloS one* 7, no. 1 (2012): e30831, https://www.ncbi.nlm.nih.gov/pmc/articles/PMC3265525/
59. Danielle McCartney et al., "Cannabidiol and Sports Performance: a Narrative Review of Relevant Evidence and Recommendations for Future Research," *Sports Medicine—Open* 6 (2020), https://www.ncbi.nlm.nih.gov/pmc/articles/PMC7338332/
60. National Academies of Sciences, Engineering, and Medicine; Health and Medicine Division; Board on Population Health and Public Health Practice; Committee on the Health Effects of Marijuana: An Evidence Review and Research Agenda, *The Health Effects of Cannabis and Cannabinoids: The Current State of Evidence and Recommendations for Research* (Washington, DC: National Academies Press, 2017), https://www.ncbi.nlm.nih.gov/books/NBK425767/

Index

About the Author

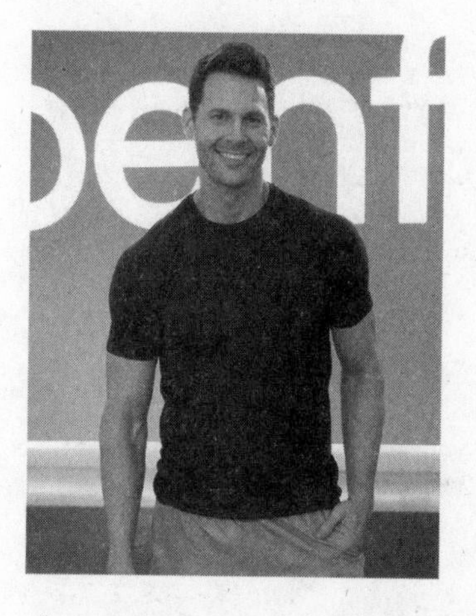

Joey Thurman is a health, fitness, and nutrition expert; consultant; and television host. He is the author of *365 Health and Fitness Hacks That Could Save Your Life* and host of *The Fad or Future Podcast*.

He was named the best trainer in Chicago by the *Chicago Sun Times*, and has appeared on countless national TV show such as *Live with Kelly and Ryan, The Today Show, Tamron Hall, Harry,* and many more. He has appeared in almost every major publication such as *Men's Health, Women's Health, PopSugar,* NPR, *NY Post, Shape, US News and World Report, Beachbody, Los Angeles Magazine*, and many more.

He is a sought-after fitness and nutrition expert getting calls to work with some of the top movie stars and celebrities in the world.

Certifications: Bachelors in Liberal Studies (BLS), Certified Personal Trainer (CPT), Corrective Exercise Specialist (CES), Fitness Nutrition Specialist (FNS), Barefoot Training Specialist (BTS), Heart Rate Performance Specialist (HRPS), Certified Stress Management Coach (CSMC), Certified Sleep Science Coach (CSSC), and Human Movement Specialist (HMS).